CARERS
Research and Practice

Edited by **Julia Twigg**

London: HMSO

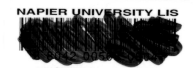

© Crown copyright 1992

Applications for reproduction should be made to HMSO
First published 1992

ISBN 0 11 701693 4

Contents

Introduction

JULIA TWIGG

Ten years ago this book could not have been written. Twenty years ago no one would have thought of writing it. Such is the measure of the changes that have overtaken informal care in the last two decades. From being a topic of marginal interest, it is now recognised as one of the lynch pins of the new community care.

How did this come about? Caring as a word only emerged in the mid 1970s. Until then the activity was scarcely visible, regarded only as an obscure and taken-for-granted aspect of family relations. Sometimes it was even assumed that families were no longer involved in this kind of activity. During the 1980s, however, the subject burgeoned academically, fuelled in large part by feminist analyses that explored the nature of caring as both labour and love, and related it to wider issues of emotional labour and women's unpaid work. Feminists were quick to point out the uneven burden of caring borne by men and women, and the degree to which community care policy rested on the unquestioned acceptance of this.

These concerns were, however, allied to others, more directly focused on the questions of community care. Much of the work on carers has concentrated on their role in supporting disabled and older people living in the community who might otherwise have to go into institutional care. This has given a particular character to the debate and to the research literature, which has tended to emphasise the prevention of institutionalisation, the cost-effectiveness of community care and the central role of carers in both. In this context, recognition of and support for carers is often justified in terms of its effectiveness as a means of supporting disabled and frail people: concern with the stress experienced by carers is presented in terms of its putative effect on their willingness to continue giving care.

These changes in academic perception have resulted in the subject moving to centre stage. It is no longer possible to ignore the involvement of carers in the support of frail and disabled people:

more severely disabled people live in the community with the help of carers than in institutions; and this is now recognised by policy makers and planners, as well as – increasingly – by politicians. In parallel with the academic understanding, therefore, has come a realisation of how common the experience of caring is within the population generally. Far from being something unusual in people's lives, caring is something that happens to many. There was some initial consternation when the Office of Population Censuses and Surveys (OPCS) data showed that upwards of six million people were involved in this activity at any one time. The figure has been much bandied about, and used in particular by pressure groups within the voluntary sector keen to see the issue achieve greater prominence. Numbers such as these, however, provoke obvious anxieties among policy makers and planners that the issue is of a size that cannot be dealt with in any but the most tokenist way. In Chapter One we try to dispel that feeling, exploring the meaning of the six million figure, and showing how it covers a range of activities and involvement. All may properly be called 'caring'; but not all require extensive service support. There are important distinctions to be made here; and the analysis presented in Chapter One should enable planners to begin to make these and to relate the policy issues they raise to the needs of their own locality. Issues concerning how agencies should respond to carers and the appropriate models they should adopt in thinking about their responsibilities are explored in Chapter Three.

It is perhaps useful at this point to add a brief note on terminology. In this book we refer to 'informal carers' – though more commonly 'carers' – and 'informal care'. The word informal is used here to distinguish it from similar care provided in the formal sector: that is provided on an organised and paid basis. Informal care by contrast normally occurs in the context of family or marital relationships, and is provided on an unpaid basis that draws on feelings of love, obligation and duty. Informal does *not* imply that the care is provided on a casual or easy going basis. Caring is often very hard work and can be emotionally draining. The term carer is sometimes used by others to mean paid staff in the 'caring' field, particular care attendants or foster carers. We avoid such use, and term these workers and their related volunteers, 'helpers'.

Caring is a generic term that embraces a range of relationships and activities. Seeing caring in this way, as something that involves a common core of experience, was very important in the emergence of the subject in the 1980s. Although many studies focused only on a particular sub–group of carers, looking at, for example, the carers of people with dementia or spouse carers, the idea of caring as a generic category that transcended such divisions grew in influence. Many of the difficulties faced by carers are common across their situations; and the impact on their lives of caring can be similar: their needs are shared ones. The generic approach was taken up by the carer lobby, reinforcing the emphasis on carers as a distinct category of people with shared needs. In this review, we encompass a range of carers: of older people, of physically disabled people, of adults with learning disabilities, and of people with mental health problems. The only significant group that has been largely excluded are the parents of disabled children of school age and younger.

Although we endorse a broadly generic approach, this needs some qualification. Although carers share many experiences, there are important differences in their circumstances and in the expectations that are made of them: being a spouse carer is not the same as caring for an elderly parent; caring for someone with dementia poses different problems from looking after someone with depression. The implications of these and other differences need to be recognised by planners and service providers. They are explored in Chapter Two.

In this book we aim to distil the lessons of research of the last decade, concentrating in particular on their relevance for practice and planning. The review has been commissioned by the Department of Health. It is intended to assist planners and practitioners in developing new responses to carers, as part of the larger changes underway in the wake of the 1990 NHS and Community Care Act. The act and the guidance associated with it emphasise the importance of carers; and responding to their needs is now recognised as central in any effective community care strategy. Over the years, the Department of Health has commissioned much research on the subject of carers, and many of the studies referred to in the following pages were funded by them. Part of the purpose of this review is to ensure that the conclusions of that body of work reach as wide an audience as possible.

In doing so we also hope – ironically perhaps for researchers and academics – to stem the tide of empirical work on this subject, and to hold back what sometimes seems like an endless stream of studies, particularly in the form of small-scale local enquiries, that do no more than repeat, often at lesser quality, findings that are already well established. We now know a great deal about the pattern and incidence of caring: of broadly who does what for whom. There is also an extensive literature on the *experience* of caring, of its burdens and stresses, as well as its more rewarding aspects. As a result, there is little to be gained from pursuing these areas further, at least at the level of the description of numbers and experiences. Local studies, though attractive to politicians and those operating in that arena, rarely reveal a different picture from that understood nationally. Caring is much the same whether undertaken in Birmingham or Bootle. It is a far more productive use of resources, particularly scarce local resources, to draw on the established literature and attempt to map its insights onto a particular locality or situation. This book aims to allow planners to do this. It also aims to inform practice and to encourage a more carer-sensitive response among service providers. To this end in Chapter Three we explore the current evidence concerning the responses of service providers to carers, drawing out some of the lessons for change. Chapter Four explores the principles that underlie effective service development, concentrating in particular on special schemes and projects.

We concentrate here on the phenomenon of caregiving and on the potential role of services in supporting carers. The focus is community care; and the services we discuss are those that are located in that sector. We do not explore the financial or economic consequences of caregiving; nor do we discuss the role of the benefit system in alleviating these. These material aspects of caring are, however, important both in understanding the situation of carers and in addressing their needs. Some at least of the problems that carers face would be alleviated if they had greater access to money that would lighten their load and enable them to purchase help. The financial and economic aspects of caring are discussed by Glendinning (1992), in her study of the financial consequences of caring, and McLaughlin (1991), in her work on the invalid care allowance (ICA).

The scope of the review has also been limited in relation to the wider circumstances of carers and the impact on them of factors such as housing, transport and employment. Caring is still largely seen as a social services issue. Caring can, however, have important consequences for people's capacity to take and sustain paid employment. Employment is also a significant source of self-esteem, as well as respite, for many carers. The last two decades have seen a growing understanding of the importance of paid work for younger women with children (though this has not gone unchallenged); and this realisation has provoked some response among employers in terms of career breaks and schemes to support women in their re-entry into the labour market. There need to be parallel developments in relation to the care of older and disabled relatives. As yet little attention has been paid at the national level within government to the questions caring raises for employment policy or legislation; and this lack of concern has been echoed among employers, with some exceptions among large organisations like the banks.

Other aspects of life also need to be seen in a caregiving context. Caring, for example, has implications for transport. The lives of many carers are unnecessarily restricted by the difficulties they face in travelling with the person they care for. They share the limitations that are imposed on disabled people generally through the inaccessibility of public buildings, the unavailability of disabled lavatories, and the hostility of the urban environment. Housing that enables the cared-for person to be as independent and self-caring as possible also helps the 'carer'; and indeed may do away with some of the need to give care. Furthermore, giving care in the context of good quality housing is very different from trying to do the same in damp, substandard housing where conditions are so crowded that the carer can never escape from the situation and have space for him or herself. Although one or two local authorities have begun to look at caring in a corporate way, as an issue that is not limited to social services but extends across the activities of the council, this is still unusual.

In the book that follows, each of the four chapters concentrates on a different aspect of caring. Gillian Parker in Chapter One draws heavily on quantitative national survey data to explore the numbers and pattern of informal carers. In doing so, she addresses the kinds of questions that planners need to consider in preparing a systematic response to the issue of informal care. Karl Atkin in Chapter Two concentrates on the differences between carers, fleshing out the experience of caring in a range of circumstances. This chapter draws more heavily on qualitative research. In Chapter Three, I discuss the potential role of mainstream services in the support of carers, concentrating on some of the evaluative work that has explored the effectiveness of various interventions. The relationship between carers and mainstream service is, however, more complex than that might imply; much of the literature on services does not fit into a simple model of evaluation but requires more complex forms of understanding. The chapter also outlines briefly some of the general issues that are raised in trying to think about the proper relationship between carers and public agencies, and consequently about the effectiveness of services in support of them. In Chapter Four, Diana Leat discusses the role of special projects and other innovative service forms, drawing out some general lessons for the management of change.

1

Counting care: numbers and types of informal carers

GILLIAN PARKER

Introduction

Recent years have seen a growing recognition of the importance of informal care. Until 1988, however, when information on informal care from the 1985 General Household Survey (GHS) was published, knowledge was patchy about the numbers and characteristics of those who support disabled and older people in the community on an informal basis. Some commentators had tried to estimate numbers by extrapolating either from national surveys of disability or from small-scale research on carers (Equal Opportunities Commission, 1982; Parker, 1985). The figures produced by this process often came out around 1.2 or 1.3 million as a minimum number of people acting as principal carers to disabled adults and children.

In 1985 the General Household Survey, a continuous national survey of adults in private households in Great Britain, for the first time asked respondents whether they were 'looking after, or providing some regular service for, someone who was sick, elderly or handicapped' either in their own household or elsewhere (Green, 1988, p. 6). This revealed a much higher number of 'carers' than previously estimated; some fourteen per cent of people aged sixteen or over said that they helped others in the way specified. Applied to the population as a whole this suggested approximately six million carers.

As might be expected, the revelation that so many people were involved in helping others to live in the community prompted substantial comment and debate. Organisations representing the views of carers were not slow to take up the figure of six million carers as a campaigning device. Even material emerging from the Department of Health's own 'Caring For People' series has treated the figure as unproblematic (Haffenden, 1991). But how useful is it for those planning and delivering services to assume that fourteen per cent of the adult population are carers?

The new community care arrangements put an explicit emphasis on population needs assessment and on the targeting of resources and, therefore, services (regardless of who is the provider) based on these assessments. Consequently, there is a real need for planners, service commissioners and providers alike to be able to take a critical look at existing population statistics such as the GHS and use them to inform their thinking.

The policy guidance from the Department of Health on implementation of the new community care 'provides the framework within which the delivery of community care should be planned, developed, commissioned and implemented locally' (Department of Health, 1990, para 1.4). As part of the planning process local authorities have the responsibility of addressing 'the needs for care services of the local population identified from a range of sources' (para 2.4). Community care plans should identify the care needs of the population 'taking into account factors such as age distribution, problems associated with living in inner city or rural areas, special needs of ethnic minority communities, the number of homeless or transient people likely to require care' (para 2.25). Further, these plans should be 'backed up by hard data, presented in an accessible way, so as to assist the identification of specific targets, and monitoring of their achievement' (para 2.28).

At the same time, the community care policy and practice guidelines put an emphasis on the needs of informal carers that has never before been articulated. They directly encourage the statutory authorities to consider the views of any informal carers when carrying out assessments of older or disabled people. Indeed, the overall provision of care is to be seen as 'a shared responsibility' between informal carers and the statutory authorities with the relationship between them seen as one of 'mutual support'. Further, 'the preferences of carers should be taken into account and their willingness to continue caring should not be assumed' (Department of Health, 1990, para 3.28).

This new emphasis means that planners and service commissioners need some idea not only of the population of people 'with care needs' but also of the population of people who are meeting those needs on an informal basis. At the same time, service providers need a clear idea of the characteristics of the population which they may be called upon to support.

These requirements present a large task of information generation and gathering. Part of the aim of this chapter is to 'short circuit' that process for informal carers, by distilling current knowledge about the numbers and types of informal carers in the population.

In this chapter we examine critically existing knowledge about the numbers and types of informal carers. The questions raised are:

- are there really six million carers?

- who are the carers?

- who are the carers most likely to need service support?

Are there really six million carers?

The GHS report itself suggests that the number of heavily involved carers may be considerably smaller than six million. Not all those who identified themselves in the GHS were principal carers; were living in the same household as the person they helped; or were caring for more than twenty hours a week (see Table 1.1). When applied to the population of Great Britain as a whole, the survey findings suggest that: 'about 1.7 million adults are spending at least 20 hours per week on providing help or supervision and about 3.7 million are bearing the main responsibility for the care of someone' (Green, 1988, p. 7).

Table 1.1   Aspects of caring situations in 1985 General Household Survey

	% of all caring relationships
Carers were sole or main carers	52
Carers lived in the same household as the person they helped	25
Carers helped for 20 or more hours a week	20
Base (100%)	3032

Large-scale surveys of disabled people have also suggested that the GHS figures may overestimate the numbers of heavily involved carers. In 1985 and 1986 the Office of Population Censuses and Surveys (OPCS) carried out a national survey of disabled adults and children, both those living in private households and those living in 'communal' settings. Adults living in private households were asked whether anyone assisted them with self-care or household activities. Fifty-six per cent of disabled adults had 'informal helpers', that is, an unpaid relative or friend who helped with any of fifteen domestic or self-care activities (Martin, White and Meltzer, 1989). The report further distinguished between 'informal carers' who helped with any of the self-care activities and 'main carers' who the disabled adults said spent most time helping them.

If the figures from the OPCS survey are applied to the total estimated population of disabled adults, a figure of 3.7 million 'informal helpers' emerges, among whom 1.2 million are 'informal carers' and, of these, 1.0 million are 'main carers'. If we add to this some estimate of the number of people acting as main carers for disabled children (assuming one for each disabled child in a private household) the final estimate for main carers becomes 1.3 million (Parker, 1990a). This figure is smaller than that suggested by the GHS but remarkably near the figures produced before the national survey was carried out.

Where do these apparent differences in estimates of the number of informal carers leave those who need to plan policy and deliver services?

Different types of caring, different types of carers
Prior to the publication of the GHS, small-scale research had suggested that the type and intensity of informal care provided, and for whom it was provided, would influence the experience of caring, and thus the need for support, in important ways. The initial report from the survey (Green, 1988) did not allow these sorts of issues to be pursued fully. Secondary analysis of the GHS data, however, has been able to pull apart the global picture of informal caring produced by the survey. A number of researchers have been involved in further analysis (for example, Arber and Ginn, 1990 and 1991; Evandrou, 1990; Parker and Lawton, forthcoming) but, inevitably, each has pursued slightly different questions in somewhat different ways. Arber and Ginn (1990, 1991 and 1992) have concerned themselves predominantly with those who support older people and have mostly distinguished between carers on the basis of whether or not they are caring for someone who lives in the same household. Evandrou (1990) has used the carer's level of responsibility for the cared-for person as a major distinguishing characteristic, while Parker and Lawton (1990a) use patterns of caring *activity* and have looked at those supporting people of all ages. Despite these differences in analysis, all the researchers have come to similar conclusions: that the 1985 GHS identified at least two different sorts of caring activity which have different implications for service planning and the provision of support.

In this section of the chapter, which concentrates on the likely numbers of informal carers who might be looking for support from service providers, we will draw largely on the programme of work carried out at the Social Policy Research Unit at the University of York and funded by the Department of Health (Parker and Lawton, forthcoming) which took caring *activities* as the basis for analysis.

Using caring activities to distinguish between carers gets away from previous research which has categorised carers in terms of who they, or those they help, are and has then gone on to describe what they do. What people do for others is likely to be influenced by who they and the person being cared for are. For example, the existing literature on informal care has suggested that the type of support provided might be influenced by whether or not the carer and the person being assisted are the same sex. Similarly, the relationship between the people involved – whether kin or not – also seems to affect the nature of assistance offered. To describe the full range of caring activity in the population, then, it is important, initially at least, to distance it from its social or relationship context.

Further, an analysis of caring activity is a useful approach if seeking recommendations for policy development or revised forms of practice to support carers. It seems more fruitful to think of providing or developing services or support on the basis of what carers *do* rather than on the basis of who they *are*. This is not to deny that the relationship between the carer and the person being cared for may influence both perceived need for support and the way in which that support might best be delivered (Twigg and Atkin, 1993). However, this approach acknowledges that knowing what carers do has a clear 'support-shaped' relevance, while knowing only who they are can imply a whole range of different levels of involvement and, therefore, needs for support.

Using the information gathered in the GHS about the types of help carers provided, Parker and Lawton (1990a) developed a 'typology' of caring activities, based on the eight tasks the GHS survey had defined:

- help with personal care, e.g. dressing, bathing, toileting

- physical help, e.g. with walking, getting in and out of bed or up and down stairs

- help with paperwork or financial matters

- other practical help, e.g. preparing meals, doing shopping, housework, household repairs

- keeping the helped person company

- taking the helped person out

- giving medicine, including giving injections, changing dressings

- keeping an eye on the helped person to see that s/he is all right.

These tasks occurred together in six quite specific patterns:
- personal *and* physical help (with or without other types of help)

- personal but not physical help (with or without other types of help)

- physical but not personal help (with or without other types of help)

- practical help with at least one other form of help *except* personal or physical

- practical help *only*

- any other combinations of help

Although some of these patterns seem rather similar, they do differentiate well between different types of carers, particularly on factors which existing research literature suggests may be associated with heavy involvement. These factors include: the hours for which carers provide assistance; whether or not anyone else helps; whether or not they share the same household as the person being helped; the number of different activities they help with; and whether or not the person they are supporting has a degree of mental impairment. Obviously, some of these factors will be closely inter-related but each one was strongly associated with helping with personal and/or physical care tasks.

Hours of caring
The GHS recorded a very wide range of involvement in caring, from people providing under two hours of help a week to those providing a hundred or more. Personal and/or physical care were highly associated with long hours of care. Some 75 per cent of those caring for between 50 and 99 hours a week and 85 per cent of those caring for over 100 hours a week were helping with personal and/or physical care (see Figure 1.1).

Figure 1.1 Type of help given by number of hours

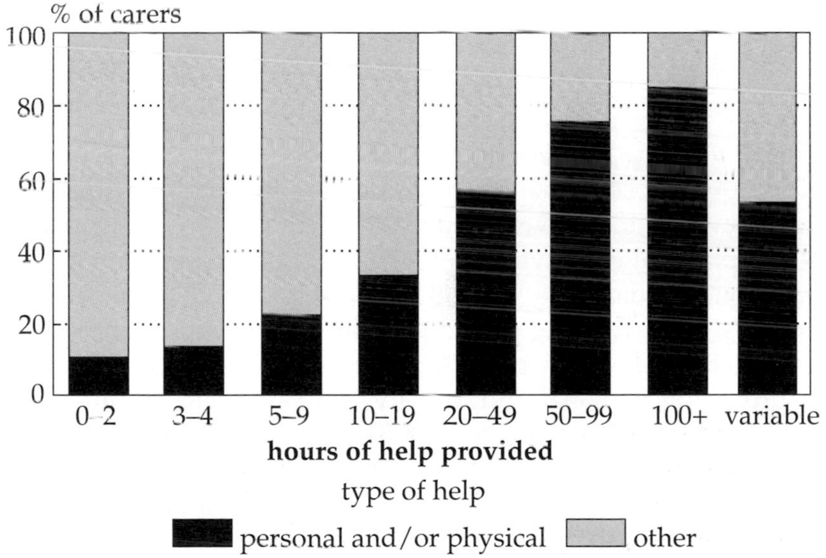

Level of responsibility

Those who identified themselves as helping someone else were asked whether or not anyone else was involved and, if so, whether that person spent more time helping than did the respondent. From answers to these questions it was possible to distinguish between sole carers; main carers (where someone else was involved but the respondent was more involved than anyone else); joint carers (where two or more people were equally involved); and 'not main carers' (where others were involved who had a greater degree of responsibility than the respondent). Those providing personal and/or physical care were almost twice as likely as others to be sole carers: 31 per cent and 19 per cent respectively (see Figure 1.2)

Figure 1.2 Level of responsibility by type of help provided

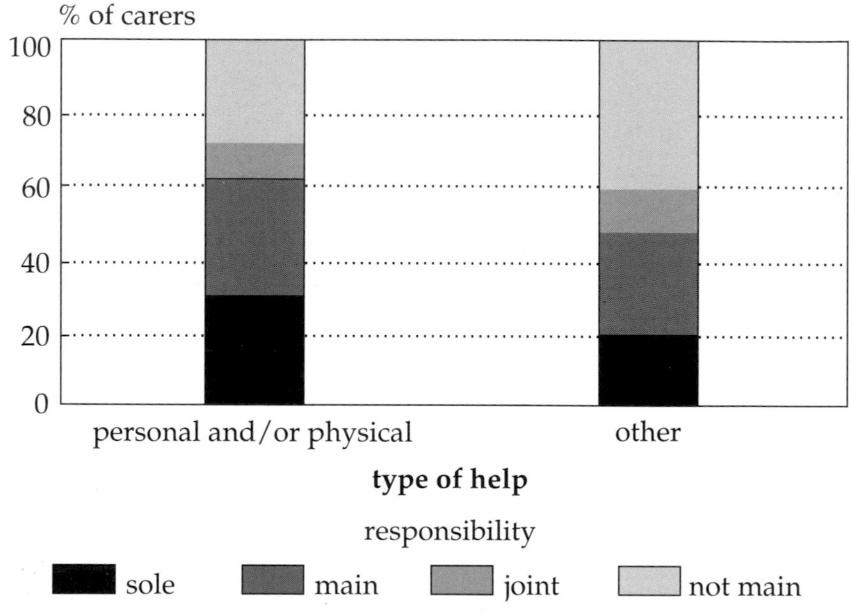

Living in the same household

The proportion of heavily involved carers helping someone in the same household was very high. Of all those providing personal and/or physical care over a half (55 per cent) were doing so in the same household as the person being helped. When personal *and* physical care were being provided some 69 per cent of carers were in the same household. By contrast, the majority (87 per cent) of those not providing personal and/or physical care were helping people who lived elsewhere (see Figure 1.3). As we shall see below, carers who live in the same household as the person they help are the least likely to be receiving any service support despite the fact that they are the most heavily involved.

Figure 1.3 Whether or not carer is in same household by type of help

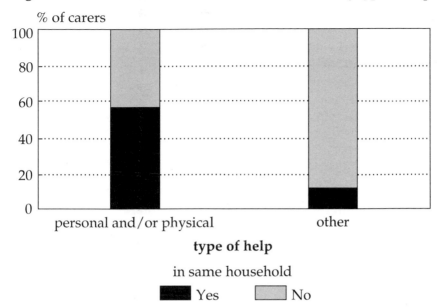

in same household

■ Yes   ☐ No

Other caring tasks
Those providing assistance with personal and/or physical tasks
were also likely to be involved in a greater number of other tasks
than were other carers. The mean task index[1] for those providing
both personal and physical care was 0.83 compared with 0.42 for
those providing 'other' help. The maximum possible task index was
1.0.

Nature of impairment
Carers in the GHS were asked what was 'wrong' with the person
they helped and how this affected them – physically, mentally or
both. The way in which the information was gathered means that it
is not possible to distinguish between people whose mental impairments are related to learning disabilities, mental health problems,
physical injuries, or degenerative conditions such as dementia.
However, individuals reported to have a degree of mental impairment were more likely to be receiving assistance with personal
and/or physical tasks. People with both physical and mental
impairments were particularly likely to be receiving personal
and/or physical help. For example, 28 per cent of carers helping
those with physical impairments only were providing personal
and/or physical care, compared to 33 per cent of those looking after

---

[1] The maximum number of tasks which any carer could be carrying out was determined by the
caring category which she or he was in. Thus, personal *and* physical care could involve all
eight tasks while 'other practical help' (see p. 10) could only ever involve a maximum of six.
The task index was calculated by dividing the number of tasks carried out by carers in each
category by the theoretical maximum for that category.

someone with mental impairments only and 45 per cent of those helping someone with both physical *and* mental impairments.

To summarise:

Any carer providing personal or physical assistance, or both, is likely to be heavily involved in that:

- they provide longer hours of help

- they are more likely to be helping with no assistance from other people

- they are looking after someone who lives in the same household

- they carry out more helping activities in total

- the person they are supporting is more likely to have some form of mental impairment.

Distinguishing between carers on the basis of the tasks they reported carrying out does seem to differentiate well between those more and less heavily involved. Helping with personal and/or physical care may be used as a proxy measure of heavy involvement with a degree of confidence, although commissioners and providers of services will need to beware of over ready or rigid use of such indicators as criteria for providing carers with support.

Analysis of this sort can also help us to move towards a more sophisticated understanding of the nature of informal care and help. On the one hand, there are people who are substantially involved, providing personal and physical care, as well as many other types of assistance, in their own household and for long hours. As we shall see below, these people are often quite elderly themselves and are most likely to be looking after a close relative. On the other hand, there is a sizeable group of people involved in activities which we might call informal *helping*. They provide practical help to friends, neighbours, and less close relatives, who do not live in the same household, and for relatively few hours. Among this second group there are some who are the only or main source of help for the other individual but, more commonly, they are part of a network where others take main responsibility.

These informal helpers play a vitally important role in helping people to live in the community. However, they are unlikely to have the same needs for close support as do those who are most heavily involved. Indeed, Arber and Ginn (1992) suggest that older people who are themselves supporting others who live elsewhere may be participating in an 'activity which is valued by the caregivers rather

14

than being perceived as a constraint on their lives' (p. 16). Further, they point out that caregiving in this group is carried out more often by people from the middle class, especially car owners. They argue that these factors may, in themselves, 'protect' carers from becoming too heavily involved.

What, then, are the likely numbers of carers in these more and less heavily involved categories? Table 1.2 outlines both the numbers and the likely percentages of adults involved in these different types of caring and helping activities.

Table 1.2　Estimates of numbers and percentages of adults in Great Britain providing help in different categories

Type of care/help	Est. numbers in GB	Est. % of adults in GB
Personal and physical	734,400	1.7
Personal not physical	559,800	1.3
Physical not personal	477,000	1.1
Practical plus	2,960,400	6.9
Practical only	453,000	1.1
Any other	815,400	1.9
Total	6,000,000	14.0

These figures should, of course, be interpreted with some caution because they can vary in either direction, both for statistical reasons and because of variation in population characteristics in any given area. For example, an area with a higher than average proportion of older people living in the community (not in residential care) is also likely to have a higher than average proportion of carers and helpers. Further, Arber and Ginn's work suggests that class (and thereby economic resources) may play an important role in determining whether or not older people in particular are able to maintain themselves independently in the community (Arber and Ginn, forthcoming). As a result, class may also be important in determining whether or not individuals become involved in caring at all and, when they do so, the level of their involvement. Consequently, the class profile of an area may also influence the numbers of heavily involved carers to be found.

Despite these provisos the re-analysed figures do indicate that the task of supporting heavily involved adult carers may be somewhat smaller than the original GHS figures might have suggested. In an 'average' area one could expect around an 'average' of four per cent of adults to be providing substantial amounts of personal and physical care to others.

15

The numbers of young children involved in care giving

The emphasis on adults in the GHS means that there is no information about the likely numbers of young children involved in caring. Over the past few years, this issue has generated much heat but relatively little light. There is no doubt that, in certain circumstances, young children do get drawn into providing care for their parents, grandparents, siblings and other relations. The Carers National Association has suggested that there may be 10,000 young carers in the country (Lunn, 1990). However, hard evidence about how many might be involved and to what extent is missing.

The GHS offers a limited opportunity to look at whether or not young adults (those who are 35 years of age or under) who have current caring responsibilities had these before the age of sixteen. In fact, some 17 per cent of these younger carers appear to have had caring responsibilities before their sixteenth birthday. Half had been helping with 'other relatives', probably grandparents, but a third had been caring for parents.

It is difficult to generalise from these figures. However, we can say that of the 1.25 million carers in the GHS who were 35 or younger, some 212,000 (17 per cent) had been caring since before the age of sixteen and, of these, around 68,000 (5 per cent) had been caring for a parent. We cannot derive any sensible population projections from these figures but they should alert us to the fact that there *are* child carers and that some of them, at least, will be heavily involved. Some of the practice issues raised by young carers are discussed in Chapter Two.

Using the figures

Although having nationally based data for the first time is extremely valuable, there are several points to make about their interpretation.

First, knowing about the numbers of people who say that they provide help to others in the community is no real guide to the 'need' for informal care. Some disabled people live without support from informal sources because of input from formal services or through packages of support which they have put together for themselves. Others may live without help from anyone else because they have housing which is suitable for their needs and have good adaptations and equipment.

This point alerts us to the ways in which the creation of disability influences the numbers of informal carers (Oliver, 1990; Morris, 1991). Personal support services, for example, may mean that disabled people do not have to rely on their family members and friends for assistance. Well-designed toilets and bathrooms may reduce the need for informal carers to be helping with aspects of personal care. Accessible transport systems may mean that disabled people can travel independently. All the factors which transform an impairment into a disability also tend to transform family members and friends into 'informal carers'. Consequently, any interventions which serve to reduce disability and 'dependence' also serve to reduce the numbers of informal carers.

A second warning about the interpretation of figures on the numbers of carers is that surveys which draw on different populations and use different questions to identify informal assistance cannot be expected to produce the same results. The two questions used in the 1985 GHS for people to identify themselves as helpers or carers were worded to be as all-inclusive in their scope as was possible. This inevitably means that some people would have identified themselves as helping individuals who would not necessarily be considered as 'disabled' by the criteria used, say, in the OPCS disability surveys. Further, as we discussed above, different definitions of 'caring' can be applied *within* surveys leading to different conclusions about 'the relative contribution of different groups to unpaid caring work' (Arber and Ginn, 1990, p. 432).

Thirdly, the OPCS survey of disabled adults asked only about help given with self-care and household activities. It may, therefore, have excluded many people who help those with mental health problems, where the main part of helping may not be the physical tasks identified in other groups (Perring *et al.*, 1990). Similarly, the GHS, with its emphasis on 'looking after or providing some regular service for', may have missed this group unless the person being supported also had some degree of physical impairment.

Finally, there is evidence to suggest that the ways in which women define themselves as 'helping' or 'caring' may have led to their under-representation in the GHS. Women may be less likely to recognise or label what they do as 'looking after' or 'special help' (Parker, 1992). This may be even more the case with 'normal' neighbourly help such as shopping, giving a lift, or calling in to keep an eye on someone. By contrast, because this behaviour is outside the bounds of what men 'normally' do, it is possible that the GHS screening question caused men to identify themselves at a level of caring activity where women would not (Arber and Ginn, 1990; Parker and Lawton, 1991b).

To summarise:

- Unquestioning acceptance of the figure of six million carers may not be helpful for planning purposes.

- There are probably around 1.3 million adult informal carers who are heavily involved in caring activities. This represents around four per cent of all adults in an 'average' area.

- The numbers of children who act as informal carers are unknown, but indications are that there may be more than previously guessed.

- The number of informal carers is not an index of the 'need' for informal care. Any interventions which reduce disability and dependence will also decrease the numbers of informal carers.

- The numbers of female carers and of those who support people with mental health problems may be underestimated in existing large-scale surveys.

Who are the carers ?

Who, then, are these people who are heavily involved in caring and likely to need support? In this section we will look at the characteristics of those providing personal or physical care, or both, at the nature of their involvement and at the characteristics of those they are helping.

Who are carers helping?

Relationship
Heavily involved carers are most likely to be looking after a spouse or a child (including an adult child). Some 75 per cent of spouse carers and 66 per cent of those helping children were involved in physical and/or personal care (Table 1.3). However, as Table 1.3 shows, whether or not the carer was helping someone in the same household was also important in determining level of involvement. This suggests that neither the relationship between the individuals involved nor the place where care takes place is enough, of itself, to indicate how heavily involved carers are to be identified.

Table 1.3 Proportion of carers providing personal/physical care in the same or a different household by relationship between carer and cared-for person

Relationship to carer	% providing personal/physical care	% providing personal/physical care in household	out of household
Spouse	72	72	0
Child	66	74	11
Parent	29	54	23
Parent-in-law	20	39	18
Other relative	25	55	19
Friend/neighbour	11	50	10

Age of person being helped
The age of the person being helped is strongly associated with the type of assistance provided, although not in the way that might be expected. Children and younger adults were the groups most likely to be being helped with personal and/or physical care tasks. Some 85 per cent of those caring for young children and 50 per cent of those helping adults aged 16 to 45 years said that they provided personal and/or physical care. By contrast, except in the very oldest age group (86 years and older) carers of older adults were less likely to be providing personal and/or physical care and more likely to be helping with practical and other tasks. Obviously one would expect young children to be more likely to be receiving help with personal care, but the results for older people are something of a challenge to received thinking about dependency in old age. However, this finding does echo information about older people generated by the 1980 and 1985 General Household Surveys which showed that it is domestic tasks, rather than personal care tasks, which present older people with problems. It also underlines recent research which demonstrates the extent to which elderly people strive to retain their independence (Wenger, 1984; Qureshi and Walker, 1989).

That the carers of older people are rather less likely to be involved in providing personal and/or physical assistance has clear implications for practice and policy in relation to domiciliary support. The informal carers of children and younger adults are the most heavily involved yet are those least likely to be receiving service support (see below).

Age of the carer
Age of the carer does not provide as sure a guide to heavy involvement in caring as other characteristics. However, those aged 56 and older were somewhat more likely than younger carers to be involved in helping with personal and physical tasks (35 per cent and 27 per cent respectively).

Sex of the carer
One of the most surprising things to emerge from the original GHS analysis was the extent to which men were involved in caring. Prior to this the literature on informal care had suggested that men were very rarely involved in providing care and that, when they were, this was in some sense aberrant (Ungerson, 1987; Dalley, 1988). By contrast, the 1985 GHS found that 12 per cent of adult men, as opposed to 15 per cent of adult women, identified themselves as carers.

We discussed earlier why men may have been more ready than women to identify themselves in this way. The original GHS analysis did show that women were more likely to be sole or main carers and to be caring for 20 or more hours a week than were men. Secondary analysis has also shown that men are rather less likely than women to be involved in the heavier forms of support. Some 32 per cent of female carers are providing assistance with personal and/or physical care compared to 26 per cent of male carers (Parker and Lawton, 1990a). Even so the findings are a considerable challenge to previous perceptions of men and informal care.

One of the reasons for these 'surprising' findings may be the nature of earlier research on informal care, which had largely concentrated on those caring for disabled children or for elderly parents living in the same household. This work showed that it was women who were most involved in caring in these situations and that it was they who bore the greatest costs. Research which concentrated on *all* older people had, however, started to show the importance of spouses as carers and, by definition, the role of male carers. For example, analysis of data on older people gathered in the 1980 GHS showed that more than 90 per cent of older married people who needed help with domestic or personal care received this from their spouse. Further, among 'severely disabled' older people living with just their spouse almost a half were women being looked after by their husbands (Arber and Gilbert, 1989).

The 1985 GHS confirmed that much of the informal care which is provided in the same household as the cared-for person is carried out by spouses, and that in such cases men and women are equally involved (Arber and Ginn, 1990 and 1991).

Further analysis (Parker and Lawton, 1991b) has tried to throw some light on the role of men as carers by addressing three different sorts of questions:

- which men are carers and how does this compare with the pattern of caring responsibility among women?

- what is the nature of caring responsibility among men compared to that of women?

- what is the impact of caring on men compared to women?

This analysis has shown that men as a group are at much less 'risk' of becoming carers. However, younger single men and older men who have ever been married are as 'at risk' as are their female peers. Co-residence is an important factor in men's caring responsibilities, suggesting that they sometimes become carers 'by default' because they have never left the parental home (Qureshi and Walker, 1989; Arber and Ginn, 1991; Glendinning, 1992).

Male carers do have a different caring profile from women; they look after different sorts of people, greater numbers of people, for somewhat shorter hours, but for longer periods. However, many of these factors are interrelated. Once we take into account the relationship between the carer and the person they are helping, and the carer's level of responsibility, few major differences between male and female carers remain. In other words, if we compare like with like we find that men and women have more similar caring profiles than previous research would have led us to believe.

The main difference which does remain between men and women, as hinted at above, is in the *type* of care that they provide. Except when they have main responsibility for the care of a spouse, men are less likely than women to be providing *personal* care. However, the nature of the relationship between the carer and the cared-for person was more influential in determining the type of care provided than was the sex of the carer.

Finally, there was little evidence to suggest that male and female carers suffered different sorts or sizes of effects on their lives as a result of caring. Both were less likely than their age/sex peers to be household heads, to be in full-time paid work, and more likely to have depressed earnings and incomes (Parker and Lawton, 1991b).

This new evidence on male caring responsibilities shows how important it is to separate out questions about the prevalence of caring responsibilities, the experiences of caring and its impact. Different answers are generated with different implications for policy and practice.

To summarise:

- With the exception of those who support people aged over 85, carers are more heavily involved when helping younger people than when helping older people.

- Age of the carer is not a good predictor of heavy involvement, although carers over the age of 55 are somewhat more heavily involved.

- Those caring for children (whether young or adult) and spouses in the same household are the most likely to be heavily involved carers.

- Although men are less likely than women to become carers, their experience of caring and its effects on their lives are not as different from those of women as previous research might have suggested. Almost the same proportion of male carers as female carers are heavily involved.

Who are the carers most likely to need service support?

As mentioned above, many of the characteristics of the heavily involved carer are interrelated. Is it possible to develop a picture of

21

the 'typical' heavily involved carer who might be the most appropriate focus for support in the new community care arrangements?

We have seen that the type of activities which carers carry out can provide a reasonable indicator of the extent to which they are heavily involved in caring, although we have also signalled that concentrating too much on practical tasks may mean that we miss the needs of those supporting people with mental health problems. By calculating the likelihood of different sorts of carers being heavily involved (as defined above) and caring for more than 20 hours a week, we can develop a 'league table' of those most likely to be in need of support. No group helping with other than personal and/or physical care and only one group helping someone in a different household with personal and/or physical tasks had odds higher than evens of providing more than 20 hours of care.

This leaves some five groups helping with personal and/or physical tasks whom one might predict would be in need of support. In descending order of the likelihood of providing more than 20 hours of care, these are:

- those caring for a child (whether or not adult) in the same household

- those caring for a spouse in the same household

- those caring for a parent in the same household

- those caring for a child in another household

- those caring for a parent-in-law in the same household

- those caring for a friend in the same household

Tasks, stress or coping?

Although the emphasis on the tasks that carers carry out, and the time they devote to caring, is useful in terms of designing and developing forms of support for them, it tells us little about the ways in which individual carers actually *cope* with their role.

One area which has attracted considerable research attention, especially in the USA, is the stress which people experience when they are caring and what factors influence this. Many researchers have produced evidence that informal carers experience increased levels of stress or emotional strain as a result of their caring responsibilities (for example, Gledhill *et al.*, 1982; Cooke, 1982; Levin *et al.*, 1989; Gilleard *et al.*, 1984; Quine and Pahl, 1885; Clarkson *et al.*, 1986; Quine and Pahl, 1989; Braithwaite, 1990).

Some might ask whether it 'matters' that informal carers experience higher levels of stress than do other members of the population. If we are concerned with questions of equity it certainly matters if some people are more stressed than others because they take responsibility for supporting disabled and older people in the community. On a more pragmatic level, it matters that carers experience high levels of stress if this means that they are less likely to be able to continue caring. Some of the policy tensions around these issues are discussed further in Chapter Three.

Evidence from studies of older, mentally infirm people does suggest that stress influences both the quality and the duration of care (Gilleard *et al.*, 1981; Levin *et al.*, 1989) and, as a corollary perhaps, drops significantly when caring ceases (Challis and Ferlie, 1988; Levin *et al.*, 1989). Although there may be important intervening variables at work between stress and the breakdown of informal care (for example, the reactions of professionals who act as 'gate-keepers' to services) it does seem that high levels of stress over a long period will affect the duration of informal caring arrangements.

For this reason alone practitioners might be looking to concentrate their attention not merely on those who carry out certain types of activity but also on those who experience these tasks as particularly stressful. As Braithwaite has pointed out:

> To assume ... that burden is the daily activities and personal care tasks provided for another is to oversimplify caregiving to the point of meaninglessness. Caregiving is a relationship between two people, and it has all the complexities of intimate human relationships. Any discussion of burden must take this into account ... To infer burden on the basis of how many tasks are being performed ... is ... tunnel-visioned ... (Braithwaite, 1990, pp. 53-4).

However, use of stress either as an indicator to intervention, or as an outcome measure after intervention, is not without its problems.

First, the experience of stress can vary both inter- and intra-personally. Two people in the same 'stressful' situation may experience quite different degrees of 'stress'. Even one individual may feel differently about similar situations at different times.

Secondly, measures of stress, for example the Malaise Inventory or the General Health Questionnaire, assume that physical or psychological symptoms parallel the 'experience' of stress. Some researchers have argued that this is not necessarily so (Hirst, 1983; Hirst and Bradshaw, 1983).

Thirdly, the experience of stress can be influenced by social or cultural factors. Expectations about what carers should or should not be expected to do may vary across time, between classes, genders and different ethnic groups, or between generations. These variations may then affect perceptions of what is or is not 'stressful'.

If stress does contribute to the breakdown of informal care, then being able to reduce stress levels may prolong it. However, successful intervention means that we need to know which *aspects* of the caring situation are causing stress and which, if any, of these factors can be improved. Here, however, research has been less than conclusive.

Much of the confusion about what causes stress in carers is due to methodological weaknesses in the research. With one or two notable exceptions there has been no attempt to take into account the inter-relationships between the variables which might cause stress, and no attempt to tie in quantitative analysis with knowledge derived from qualitative work on caring. Thus the inter-relationships between age and sex of the carer, sex and level of dependency of the person being helped, and the kin relationship between them are rarely considered, when qualitative work has suggested that, in combination, these interactions are likely to be very important in the mediation of stress.

There are some areas in which existing research on the carers of older people, especially of those with mental impairments, does agree. Broadly speaking, it seems that 'demand' on the carer – the demands on the attention and emotions of the carers that older infirm people make, such as disrupting the carer's social life, always asking questions, demanding attention, creating personality clashes – contributes most to reported levels of strain (Gilleard *et al.*, 1984; Levin *et al.*, 1989). However, there is little agreement in the research literature about the factors associated with raised levels of stress among those supporting older people more generally, younger adults or children.

Recently a number of commentators have started to question whether the search for 'predictors' of stress is a useful one (Byrne and Cunningham, 1985; Zarit, 1989). As argued above, with the limited exception of those looking after mentally infirm older people, it has proved difficult to come to any conclusion, however tentative, about what may 'cause' high levels of stress in carers. Carers undoubtedly do experience higher levels of stress than the general population, as measured on the available scales and tests, yet the intuitively plausible reasons why this might be so (nature and degree of impairment, the extent to which the cared-for person has to depend on the carer, low self-care skills, and so on) appear to offer no convincing explanation. Given the contradictions in what has been found, then, why continue the pursuit?

In fact, more promising avenues may be opened up by approaching the issue from a different angle. Given that carers experience more stress than is the norm, and given that the nature and degree of impairment, and for some at least, the extent of disability, are immutable, does it make more sense to direct attention to those factors which help carers to 'cope' or which *reduce* stress levels? (Byrne and Cunningham, 1985; Parker, 1985 and 1990; Titterton, 1992.)

In fact the research literature already contains suggestions that there are aspects of carers' lives which help them to cope. Three major factors emerge as particularly important: time off from caring, satisfaction with help from others, and receipt of services.

i   Time off from caring

One of the most significant factors in reducing stress levels in carers may be time away from the person being cared for, whether because the carer can get out or because the person being supported can. This applies to carers of older people as much as it does to those helping younger adults or children (Thompson and Haran, 1985; Hirst, 1984; Levin *et al.*, 1989). For younger carers, particularly the mothers of disabled children, being able to go to work has a very strong protective effect against stress (Bradshaw and Lawton, 1976; Hirst, 1984).

Only two per cent of the carers in the GHS who were helping someone in the same household reported that the cared-for person spent time away from home, whether with friends of relatives or in some type of residential setting (Green, 1988). Further, in fewer than a third of cases did the cared-for person attend work, school, college or any form of social activity during the day. The older the person being cared for was, the less likely it was that he or she would be involved in any form of day-time activity outside the home.

Arranging a two-day break caused much greater problems for all carers and appeared to be almost impossible for those who were heavily involved. Almost half of those looking after someone in the same household said that no one else could look after the cared-for person, and another fifth said that it would be fairly or very difficult to arrange alternative care (Green, 1988). Again, heavily burdened carers were in an even more difficult position.

As a result of the difficulty of arranging alternative care, more than half of carers looking after someone in the same household had not had a break of at least two days since they started caring (Green, 1988). Those looking after adult offspring were most likely to report problems arranging a two-hour absence, explained in part by the relatively high proportion of these 'same household' carers who were looking after someone with a mental impairment. Spouse carers, by contrast, were the ones who found it most difficult to arrange a two-day break. Of all 'same household' carers, spouses were the ones least likely to have had a break of two days since starting caring (70 per cent), followed by those looking after a young child (55 per cent), those looking after an adult child (50 per cent), and those caring for a parent (43 per cent).

Another way in which carers can be said to get 'time off' from caring is when *they* have some activity outside the home. In fact, among all carers, half were without day-time activity (whether paid work, education or training) which would have taken them out of the home. For the most heavily involved this proportion rose to 59 per cent, and among the most heavily involved who were looking after someone in the same household to 68 per cent.

Among people under pensionable age carers were less likely to be in paid work than their peers. Again, the more heavily involved the carers were the less likely they were to be in paid work. Similarly, caring for someone in the same household reduced the likelihood of being in paid employment, and particularly so for women (Parker and Lawton, 1990b).

Participation in paid work also varied substantially with the age of the cared-for person. Those helping older people were more likely than any other group of carers to have retired. However, working-age carers of older people were more likely than any other group of working age carers to be in some form of paid employment, as Table 1.4 shows. By contrast, women caring for younger children were substantially less likely than other women of working age to be in paid employment (Baldwin and Parker, 1991).

Table 1.4   Proportion of male and female carers of working age in paid work by age of cared-for person and type of care provided

Age of cared for person	% male carers in paid work	in same household	not	% female carers in paid work	in same household	not
0–15 years	68	67	100	31	28	67
16–45 years	57	58	54	44	41	47
46–65 years	64	54	71	54	48	56
66–75 years	75	78	75	61	55	61
76+ years	75	56	79	61	63	61
All	72	61	76	58	48	60

In sum, paid employment does not offer any substantial 'respite' to the most heavily involved carers, even for those for whom it might reduce stress rather than adding to their role overload.

ii   *Help from others*

Neither the measurement of help given to main carers by other informal helpers, nor the subsequent analysis of this information, has been very sophisticated. Evidence about the relationship between the *amount* of help given and reductions in carers' stress is consequently equivocal. However, studies do repeatedly show that when carers are happy with the amount of help they get from others, regardless of how much that actually is, stress is reduced. Again, this effect is evident among carers involved with different groups of disabled or older people (Nissel and Bonnerjea, 1982; Glendinning, 1983; Gilhooly, 1986).

Contacts with others provide the opportunity for more than just practical help, of course; intimacy, confiding relationships and emotional help may also be available. The scope for being helped by others in any of these ways is related to the extent of social support which the carer has more generally. Given that caring and disability often lead to reduced social networks (Parker, 1992), any interventions which help carers and those they assist to maintain their networks will be important.

As we saw earlier there is little to suggest that the most heavily involved carers are particularly assisted by others. First, these carers are more likely to be caring alone than are others. Secondly, heavily involved carers living in the same household as the person they support are more likely than others to live in two-person households.

iii *Provision of services*
We discuss the role of services in reducing the stress of carers in greater detail in Chapters Three and Four. It is worth pointing out here that certain types of service receipt have been associated with reduced levels of stress in principal carers. Domiciliary support in particular, for example visits from home helps and community nurses, appears to help those caring for elderly, mentally infirm people to cope (Levin *et al.*, 1989; Gilhooly, 1984). Despite this, however, no service intervention seems as effective at reducing stress levels for those caring for older, mentally infirm people, as does entry of the older person into residential or hospital care (Levin *et al.*, 1983; Challis and Ferlie, 1988).

Early, small-scale research on informal care suggested that service provision essentially served to support older and disabled people who lived alone and rarely to support or replace informal carers. Larger-scale data on older people suggested not only that services primarily supported those living alone, but that service receipt for older people who lived with others was influenced by the type of household in which they lived (Arber *et al.*, 1988).

The 1985 GHS also seemed to suggest that services were more likely to go to those without resident carers. People whose carers live in a different household are twice as likely to receive regular visits from their GP or a social worker, four times as likely to have a home help, and ten times as likely to receive meals-on-wheels as those whose carers are in the same household (Green, 1988). There was little difference, however, in levels of contact with community or district nurses.

At first sight, it seems that this imbalance in the provision of services might be due to the greater proportion of people whose carer lived elsewhere and who themselves lived alone. However, further analysis of the GHS data suggests otherwise (Parker and Lawton, 1991a).

With the exception of the meals-on-wheels service, initial analysis suggests that all services were relatively 'well-targeted' in relation to the type of help which the main carer was providing. In other words, if there were no other differences between people, we would find that services were going to those whose main carers were the most heavily involved. However, there *are* differences between people, both in their relationship to the carer and in whether or not they live in the same household.

Multi-variate analysis makes it possible to control for the likely interactions between such factors as: the age of the person being cared for; the level of assistance which his or her informal carer provides; and his or her relationship to the carer. Analysis of this sort showed that these factors were far more important in determining service provision than was the extent to which the carer was heavily involved. Those being cared for by relatives in the same household were, across the board, less likely to be receiving services than others. Moreover, some services appeared to discriminate more against some categories of carers than others. The home help service, for example, was the one least likely to be going to those cared for by relatives in the same household, regardless of how heavily involved the main carer was. By contrast, community nursing services appeared to be delivered more equitably than others. The analysis also tried to tease out the effect of living alone, to see if this accounted for the greater receipt of services among those whose carers lived elsewhere, but came to the conclusion that it did not (Parker and Lawton, 1991a).

The GHS did not 'measure' stress, as such. However, by looking at the factors identified above as being possible stress *reducers* and seeing to what extent they are present in the lives of those we defined earlier as 'heavily burdened', we can see that the carers who, from first principles, should be the ones receiving most support are actually the ones least likely to be doing so.

To summarise:
- Although informal carers experience a higher level of stress than the population at large, there are few clear indicators to the specific factors which cause increased stress.

- A more useful approach may be to think about the factors which help carers to 'cope'.

- Factors which do seem to help carers to cope are: time off from caring; satisfaction with help from others in their informal network; and services receipt.

- Heavily involved carers are unlikely to be able to take 'time off' from caring, whether through day-time activity for themselves or for the person they support.

- There is no evidence that heavily involved carers are more likely than others to receive help from informal sources.

- Existing patterns of service receipt appear to discriminate against those caring for relatives who live with them, yet these are the very groups who are most heavily involved in caring.

2

Similarities and differences between informal carers

KARL ATKIN

Introduction

Over the past ten years generic approaches to informal care have dominated policy debates. The 'burdens' and restrictions faced by carers as well as their needs for practical support and regular breaks have been seen as features common to the experience of all carers. This approach, although important in gaining recognition for carers as a group, does not adequately reflect some of the significant differences between carers. These differences need to be recognised if appropriate services are to be developed. This chapter concentrates on three important areas of difference: the relationship between the carer and the person they look after; the disability of the cared-for person; and more general aspects of the carers' backgrounds.

Relationships

The nature of the relationship affects the experience of care and what carers do as well as the response of service practitioners. The implications of this will be examined in more detail by exploring six different forms of caring relationship: spouse carers, parental carers, filial carers, sibling carers, child carers, and non-kin carers.

Spouse carers
Two specific expectations govern informal care within spouse relationships. First, the care given by spouse carers is often seen as an extension of the love and support that is a mutual expectation of modern marriage. Not to give such care would seem to deny the very basis of marriage. Secondly, the assumption of being and remaining together is implicit in marital relationships. These expectations mean that the support given by spouse carers is often taken for granted by

service practitioners. Evidence suggests that of all caring relationships spouse carers are the least likely to have outside help (Green, 1988).

Although there is an expectation that spouses will provide continuing care for their disabled husband or wife, they face particular problems in doing so. First, spouse carers do not enter marriage expecting to provide intimate physical care and doing so challenges their 'normal' expectations (Parker, 1992). Service practitioners should not make assumptions about the easy extension of marital intimacy into other forms of physical intimacy. Secondly, impairments associated with changed behaviour or personality are very stressful for spouse carers (Rosenbaum and Najenson, 1976; Oddy *et al.*, 1978; Kinsella and Duffy, 1979; Gilhooly, 1984). Carers feel a particular sense of loss because of the transformation these changes can cause in the relationship.

Thirdly, carers often face a limited social life as a result of the inability of their husband or wife to share in it (Parker, 1992; Twigg and Atkin, 1993); and this creates a series of dilemmas for spouse carers. Spouse carers often want to get away from the other person's company, yet the person they most want to go out with is their spouse. Carers often experience guilt about enjoying themselves when the person they love cannot. The expectations implicit in marital relationships make it difficult for the carer to articulate a need for an independent social life; wanting respite may seem disloyal and threaten the basis of married life. Building up a separate social life may seem to undermine the relationship, yet, at the same time, constantly being in each other's company creates enormous strains. These carers, therefore, face considerable difficulties in pursuing a social life.

Fourthly, as with all carers, caring has an impact on the financial resources and labour market participation of spouse carers (Joshi, 1987; Martin and White, 1988; Glendinning, 1992). In households where a spouse becomes disabled, carers of working age may experience a sudden change in circumstances which makes it impossible for them to continue working (Parker, 1990). Indeed having a disabled spouse reduces the likelihood of the carer being in paid work. This can be further compounded by the additional costs of having a disabled person in the household. Such households face the double disadvantage of extra needs but few resources to meet them. Evidence suggests that service practitioners can make this disadvantage more severe than it need be, and reduce the ability of the carer to work by failing to provide help with domiciliary and personal care tasks, or allocating day time respite (Blaxter, 1976).

To summarise:
- It is often taken for granted by service practitioners that spouse carers will care for a disabled husband or wife. Expectations of marital life serve to enforce this.

- Spouse carers experience difficulties in coping and coming to terms with their husband or wife especially when this is associated with changed behaviour or personality.

- Service practitioners should not assume spouse carers find it easy to undertake tasks involving physical intimacy.

- Carers often find it difficult to articulate their experience of the restrictions on their social life. Service practitioners must recognise dilemmas that arise in relation to this.

- Looking after a spouse affects the ability of the carer to work. The financial impact of this is compounded by the extra costs associated with having a disabled person in the household.

Parental carers

Although there is an element of choice for an adult child in deciding to care for their mother or father, society rarely sanctions the same degree of choice for a parent with regard to her or his children (Parker, 1990). Parental carers, although expected to care, face a number of difficulties which can continue even when their child reaches adulthood. These include physical care tasks, the emotional 'burdens' of caring, as well as the impact on financial resources and labour market participation.

The 'daily grind' of caring for a disabled child is well documented (Bayley, 1973; Wilkin, 1979; Glendinning, 1983; Baldwin, 1985). In addition, however, there are the emotional costs associated with coming to terms with the child's disability and balancing the needs of other family members. Parents often experience considerable difficulties in coming to terms with their child's disability, especially if that disability arises from a severe intellectual impairment. Carers can experience a range of emotions such as guilt, frustration, anxiety and resentment, and many need help in coming to terms with the birth of a disabled child (Bayley, 1973; Wilkin, 1979; Chetwynd, 1985; Quine and Pahl, 1985). Moreover, these feelings are not confined to the immediate period after birth but can occur, in varying degrees, throughout childhood, even continuing after the child reaches adulthood. Service practitioners have an important role to play in helping carers to cope and come to terms with their child's disability, and need to offer this support on both an occasional and long-term basis. In addition, carers often worry that they are neglecting their spouse and other children by concentrating on the needs of the disabled offspring. Attempting to strike a balance can prove stressful, particularly for mothers (Burton, 1975; Carr, 1976; Wilkin, 1979; Glendinning, 1983).

An important feature of parental carers is the different caring responsibilities of mother and father. Mothers usually have a greater involvement in the care of disabled offspring than fathers; and each tends to carry out different tasks (Bayley, 1973; Burton, 1975; Carr, 1976; Wilkin, 1979; Glendinning, 1983 and 1985). Fathers, for example, tend to provide help with the more pleasurable activities: whereas mothers have responsibility for the intimate day-to-day caring tasks. The care is not shared equally.

Caring for a disabled child affects labour market participation of both mother and father, but in different ways. Both face restrictions on their choice of employment and promotion opportunities. Furthermore, evidence suggests that looking after a disabled child has considerably more impact on the mother's employment opportunities by restricting her ability to work outside the home (Burton, 1975; Wilkin, 1979; Baldwin and Glendinning, 1983; Hirst, 1985 and 1992; Smyth and Robus, 1989). Clear evidence of the effect on the mother's employment opportunities of caring for a child with severe disabilities is provided by Bradshaw's (1980) study of Family Fund applicants. Among families applying, only 24 per cent included mothers who were in paid employment outside the home, compared to 41 per cent of families in the General Household Survey for a comparable year. Although almost a quarter of the fathers reported that their employment had been adversely effected by their child's disability, they tended to miss hours and days at work rather than give up or lose jobs altogether.

Inability to participate fully in the labour market can have a considerable impact on the family's earnings. Average gross earnings for all people with children are 9 per cent higher for men and 7 per cent higher for women than those found among parents with disabled children (Smith and Robus, 1989). Loss of earnings, however, is only one aspect of the financial cost of caring for a disabled child, and is compounded by the fact that day-to-day living expenses are likely to be higher (Hyman, 1982; Baldwin, 1985). Research suggests that 90 per cent of families with a disabled child had extra costs associated with disability (Baldwin, 1985). Causes of extra expenditure included: clothes, bedding, extra laundry, heating, transport costs, special food and diets, housing and house adaptations, repairs to house and furniture, and aids to mobility and daily living.

The difficulties facing parental carers continue when the child reaches adulthood (Hirst, 1985, 1992). Parental carers of disabled adults, however, face another set of difficulties as a consequence of their child's transition to adulthood (Sines and Bicknell, 1985; Race, 1987; Twigg and Atkin, 1993). Leaving home, getting a job, having a private sexual life are seen as significant in achieving adulthood and independent living. Many parental carers, although wanting to encourage greater independence, feel threatened by these changes and uncertain about their own position (Further Education Unit, 1990; Twigg and Atkin, 1993).

The carers' relationship with service practitioners reflects some of these concerns. Parental carers, for example, can feel that service practitioners adopt an unrealistic view of the cared-for person's ability and this annoys and frustrates them; on the other hand service practitioners frequently describe carers as being over-protective and not recognising the full potential of the person they care for. Parental carers, in particular, see the transition to adulthood as an enormous risk, with services not having sufficient resources to achieve full independent living for their child (Twigg and Atkin, 1993).

Securing an acceptable future provision for their child after their own death is another worry for parental carers (Ineichen *et al.*, 1980; Hirst, 1985; Twigg and Atkin, 1993). This represents a particularly upsetting subject, especially when they see what they perceive as the failures of community care policy around them. Carers, having seen people diagnosed as mentally ill wandering the streets, fear that will happen to their offspring (Twigg and Atkin, 1993). Carers' anxieties about future provision also include the type of caring arrangements that will be offered to their child as well as concerns about financial provision (Jones, 1988; Twigg and Atkin, 1993). Carers, for example, often have preferences for particular types of accommodation such as small hostels with a permanent care worker attached. The fact that these preferences sometimes conflict with current service philosophies adds to their worries.

Finally, there is the general issue of 'visibility'. Carers of disabled children are likely to be known to service practitioners. For a series of bureaucratic and administrative reasons there is greater surveillance of children than adults, and consequently any child with a disability should be known to service practitioners. In particular the child's contact with educational institutions ensures they are visible. It should not be assumed, however, that this visibility is carried through to adult life. As disabled children leave school, there is a possibility that they will become 'lost' to services (Hirst, 1985). Some carers, for example, feel that once their child reaches adulthood he or she will receive less support.

To summarise:

- Parental carers often have to balance the needs of the disabled child with those of other family members and this can be a considerable source of stress.

- Mothers usually have a greater involvement in the care of disabled offspring than fathers.

- The labour market participation of parental carers is restricted by caring and the impact of this is greater for women. Caring for a disabled child also has important financial consequences and daily living expenses are likely to be greater than those of a family without disabled offspring.

- Parental carers worry about securing acceptable future provision for their offspring after their own death. Service practitioners need to discuss future options carefully.

- Carers often experience anxiety during the child's transition to adulthood. Service practitioners need to be sensitive to this and be aware of the importance of offering continuing support.

Filial carers

Past literature suggests that offspring, and especially daughters and daughters-in-law, are the mainstay of informal care. Although recent evidence demonstrates the importance of spouse carers, it remains the case that where there is no husband or wife available, care usually falls to a member of the immediate family, and in particular to a daughter or daughter-in-law (Qureshi and Walker, 1989).

The relationship between child and parent sets up a different set of expectations than in other kin relationships. What is acceptable and expected for a parent to do for a child is very different from what a child might do for a parent. The performance of tasks involving physical intimacy, for example, is less likely to be seen as an accepted part of an adult daughter's or son's relationship with their parent (Lewis and Meredith, 1988); whereas for parents it is a customary part of their relationship with younger offspring. A filial carer's relationship with their parent also differs from a spouse relationship. Not only is the obligation to care less binding among filial carers but there is a greater tradition of independence between a daughter or son and their disabled parent. Each has established separate lives before the need for care arises (Parker, 1992; Twigg and Atkin, 1992). Furthermore it should not be assumed because the carer looks after their mother or father that they enjoy a close relationship. The caring relationship between mother and daughter, for example, has been described as being fraught with ambivalence (Lewis and Meredith, 1988). Indeed some relationships can become less close as a result of caring.

Filial carers fall into two general categories: those who share a household with their parents and those who do not. Among those who share a household, there is in turn a distinction to be made between those who have never left home or who have moved back in the wake of marital separation, and those who have set up a joint household specifically in order to care for their elderly parent. Among the first group, there is rarely a conscious decision to care, and these individuals tend to drift into the role. This pattern is particularly characteristic of sons (Ungerson, 1987; Lewis and Meredith, 1987). Those carers who live in the same household as the cared-for person are more likely to undertake greater caring responsibility than out-of-household carers, particularly in relation to physical tending (Lewis and Meredith, 1988). Becoming a carer can create particular difficulties for this group. They can find it difficult to go out, see family or friends or go on holiday; this can be particularly frustrating since the carer being single or divorced is likely to have expectations of an independent personal and social life. These carers may also have considerable anxieties about the future. The length of time they will have to care remains uncertain, and, therefore, they find it difficult to plan. Once the cared-for person has died, carers experience loneliness and loss of purpose and usually require help and support in coming to terms with their bereavement (Lewis and Meredith, 1988; Levin et al., 1989).

Some shared households are formed specifically in order to give care, with the carer either moving in with his or her elderly parents or, more commonly, with the elderly parents coming to share the home of his or her son or daughter. The period directly following a move represents an important transitionary stage in the relationship and help may be required as child and parent adjust to the new living arrangement.

Perhaps the biggest difficulty facing filial carers is that of balancing their family and social responsibilities with caring for their parent or parent-in-law. This can be made harder if the carer needs to travel constantly between two homes (Wenger, 1984; Sinclair, 1990). Balancing these competing claims on their time can become stressful.

The expectations that characterise the relationship between child and parent are evident in the response of service practitioners. Service practitioners tend to regard a son's or daughter's relationship with their parent as less private than that between wife and husband (Parker, 1992; Twigg and Atkin, 1993). This can mean they are more willing to 'intrude' on the relationship and to offer certain forms of support. This can be illustrated with reference to the carer's need for a social life. Encouraging and enabling a spouse to pursue an independent social life can, as we have seen, create tensions for service practitioners as well as carers. Maintaining an independent social life for a filial carer is often viewed as a more legitimate use of service resources. Service practitioners tend in these cases to recognise the competing claims of the carer's other relationships (Twigg and Atkin, 1993). The breakdown of care provides another example of different expectations in regard to relationships. Since the obligation to care tends to be less binding among filial carers than spouse carers, the end of caregiving is open to greater negotiation (Twigg and Atkin, 1993). Service providers are more prepared to support the carers in deciding to give up care, particularly if they feel that caring is becoming detrimental to their well-being.

It would be misleading, however, to say that filial carers receive extensive support. The problems they face in getting help are similar to other carers. Their involvement is often taken for granted by service practitioners, and they face difficulties in getting their needs recognised. Moreover, service practitioners often assume that a disabled person's children will automatically provide help, without considering their other responsibilities.

To summarise:

- When a spouse is not available to care for his or her husband or wife, that caring responsibility usually falls to offspring.

- Balancing the demands of other family responsibilities can prove stressful for many carers.

- Carers face an uncertain future and do not know how long they will need to care. Planning for the future can, therefore, be difficult.

- Service practitioners often assume that offspring will automatically provide help, without considering their other responsibilities.

Sibling carers

There is little information describing the experience of siblings as carers. Some authors go as far as to suggest that sibling relationships are relatively unimportant in discussions about informal care (Lee and Ihinger-Tallman, 1980). Although the number of sibling carers providing informal care is less than three per cent of the total number of carers (Green, 1988), their contribution should not be overlooked (Kivett and Maxheamer, 1980; Wenger, 1984; Wright, 1986).

Siblings offer care in a variety of circumstances. First, there are school-age children, still living at home, who help out their parents in the care of a disabled brother or sister. These 'carers' do not usually undertake the main responsibility for care, but are on hand to help their parents This may including playing with their sibling, as well as keeping an occasional eye on him or her (Glendinning, 1983 and 1985). For these younger carers it is sharing a household with a disabled sibling that has a greater impact on their lives. Siblings, for example, may have to accommodate challenging behaviour if their brother or sister has a learning disability. In addition non-disabled siblings can also experience disadvantage, as parents not only give more time to their disabled brother or sister, but also because the household has more limited financial resources caused by the extra costs of caring for a disabled child (Quine and Pahl, 1985). Children can, for example, feel unsupported at school or be unable to go out on day trips with friends because their parents can not afford the cost. Having a disabled child in the family can create potential tensions within the family, with the non-disabled siblings feeling neglected. This can continue into adult life, raising the possibility of a poor relationship between siblings. This is particularly common when one sibling is diagnosed as mentally ill, and can have important implications for relationships within the family (Twigg and Atkin, 1993), with parents often feeling they are caught in the middle.

Secondly, there are those siblings who offer support to parents after they have left home. This support usually takes the form of emotional support and rarely includes help with physical tasks (Wenger, 1984; Wright, 1986). Parents, for example, will often seek their advice (Twigg and Atkin, 1993). Many parental carers, however, are reluctant to turn to their children for help with more physical and personal care tasks. They feel it is unfair to expect their children to help, particularly when they have family obligations of their own (Qureshi, 1986; Sinclair et al., 1988; Twigg and Atkin, 1993). Service practitioners should not assume that parents will share the caring responsibility with their adult children.

Occasionally siblings assume care for a disabled brother or sister after the death of a parent. Nowadays most parents do not seem to expect their children to care for their siblings. Twenty years ago, however, this was often the preferred option, particularly when the only alternative was a 'subnormality' hospital; and it was usually the oldest daughter who took on the responsibility. This, although rare, still occurs today. These carers have usually been caring for a considerable length of time and share certain similarities with parental carers. Consequently they often share similar concerns about the transition to independent living, as well as being anxious about future provision if anything were to happen to them.

Fourthly, there are those siblings who have never established a separate household from their brother or sister and who in time become carers by virtue of sharing the household (Wenger, 1984). These are usually elderly siblings. As with filial carers who have never left home, these individuals often become carers without realising it. These sibling carers also share other similarities with filial carers. Balancing their social and personal lives with their caring responsibilities, for example, can prove stressful. These carers have usually established a social life independent of their sibling and as the demands of caring increase the carer can find her/his social life being slowly eroded.

Finally, in rare cases older people may move in with siblings following the death of their partner. This is often for companionship but may later develop into mutual care.

To summarise:

- There is little information describing the experience of siblings as carers and their contribution to community care, while limited, is often overlooked.

- Parents are reluctant to turn to their children for help, particularly when their children have family obligations of their own. Service practitioners, therefore, should not assume that parents will share the caring responsibility with their adult children.

Child carers

As we have seen in the previous chapter, estimates suggest there are 10,000 informal carers under the age of 16 (Sandwell, 1989; Tameside, 1989). They usually provide care in single parent families in which the parent develops a disabling illness. Other examples of young carers occur with children living with an older grandparent or, as we have seen, where older children help out with the care of a disabled sibling.

Children's caring responsibility can have a serious effect on their personal and educational development (Sandwell, 1989; Meredith, 1990; Hills, 1991). Poor school attendance is common and it is estimated that a third under-attain educationally. Moreover, as well as the physical side of caring, evidence suggests that the emotional pressures of caring can lead to difficulties in forming social relationships. Many child carers, for example, find they cannot participate in the same activities as their friends because of caring responsibilities and consequently feel isolated.

Despite these problems, young carers sometimes face difficulties in being recognised by service practitioners (Meredith, 1989; Hills, 1991). First, children are not expected to provide this sort of care and as a result are often not identified as doing so by service practitioners. Secondly, even where children are identified as carers they will often deny it out of fear and loyalty, as caring is not a part of the expected relationship between parent and child. Thirdly, parents and children are often unwilling to let practitioners know they need help because they fear that their child may be taken into care.

Not surprisingly intervention by service practitioners in these situations is particularly sensitive because of the danger of breaking up the family (Hills, 1991). Practitioners must recognise the reluctance of the family for the child to be identified as a carer. Reassuring the cared-for person that their child will not be taken into care is an important starting point.

To summarise:

- A significant amount of informal care is provided by people under the age of 16 and caring can have a serious effect on their personal and educational development.

- Young carers often remain hidden from service providers.

- Service practitioners need to offer reassurance to overcome the reluctance of families to identify children as carers. A particular fear is the possibility that the child may be taken into care.

Non-kin carers

Friends and neighbours are sometimes presented as the bedrock of care in the community (Griffiths, 1988). Their role as principal carers, however, appears to be limited (Wenger, 1984; Green, 1988; Hills, 1991). The help they provide has been characterised as 'infrequent practical help' and usually concerns general social aspects of care such as sitting, providing transport, and help with shopping, often in response to minor problems and crises in everyday life (Bayley, 1973; Wilmot, 1987; Sinclair, 1990). As a general rule non-kin carers are not involved in intimate or physical care. Indeed offering emotional support to the principal carer is the main form of help given by non-kin carers. Many older people prefer to talk to friends rather than their children (Lewis *et al.*, 1989), as they feel their children are 'too closely involved'. Friends can also provide essential encouragement to the carer, and occasionally this has been identified as a vital aspect in the continuation of care (Twigg and Atkin, 1993).

In general people want neighbours and friends on hand but not in 'the front room' (Sinclair, 1990; Hills, 1991). For their part neighbours and friends are usually happy to lend a hand in an emergency or when they can do so without too much disruption to their own lives. They are wary of taking on long-term commitments. They also have less of an obligation to care than kin carers and find it easier to give up their role, especially if too much is expected of them. The involvement of these carers needs to be respected but not taken for granted.

To summarise:

- The role of non-kin carers is usually limited to tasks such as sitting, providing transport, and help with shopping. There is rarely much involvement in intimate or physical care.

- Non-kin carers have less of an obligation to care in comparison to kin carers, and service practitioners should not take their involvement for granted.

The disability of the cared-for person

This section will examine the consequences for informal care of four categories of disability: physical disability, learning disability, those experiencing mental health problems, and disability among older people.

Physical disability

Physical disabilities affect young and older people and cover a wide range of conditions, each having different consequences for the carer. The role of these carers, although varied, has common aspects that affect the relevance of service provision and the usefulness of subsequent intervention. People with a physical disability often need help with bathing, dressing, getting in and out of bed, lifting, and toileting, as well as with household activities (Glendinning, 1983; Nissel and Bonnerjea, 1982; Lewis and Meredith, 1988; Parker, 1992). These carers often face a physically demanding role and support with these tasks, in which services substitute for the carer, is much valued. Carers, however, identify problems of timing (Twigg and Atkin, 1993). These tasks, by their nature, have to be performed at specific times and service practitioners find it difficult to guarantee this.

Carers' involvement with physical care tasks is not necessarily limited to the direct performance of them; some carers supervise the cared-for person in personal and physical care tasks and are on hand if they require help (Lewis and Meredith, 1988; Twigg and Atkin, 1993). A person with arthritis, for example, may be able to bath but need help getting out of the bath. Some carers also like to keep an eye on the person they care for, in case their help is required. They might want to make sure the person does not slip in the bath or fall when getting out of bed. In this sense these carers assume a degree of responsibility for the person they look after. Service practitioners, however, often see appropriate support to carers only in terms of support with physical tasks and overlook the other difficulties faced by these carers.

The onset of disability can be a time of considerable stress for the carer (Byrne and White, 1983). Carers not only have to come to terms with a new role, but also with a person restricted by disability. The carer's world, in effect, is turned upside down (Parker, 1992) and this is especially true if the disability occurs without warning, as a result of, say, a car or industrial accident. Other conditions resulting in physical impairment, such as chronic illness where onset is more gradual, create a different set of problems for the carer. First, these disabilities can be episodic in character. This is particularly true of conditions such as multiple sclerosis, sickle cell disease, and rheumatoid arthritis, where the sufferer may experience times of crisis interspersed with periods of relative stability. This requires a much more flexible response and service practitioners need to be prepared to vary their response accordingly; carers may continue for long periods without needing help and then need immediate help at the onset of a crisis. Secondly, the possibility of long-term decline means that these carers face a greater degree of uncertainty about how the cared-for person's disability will affect their lives (Falek, 1979; Action for Research into Multiple Sclerosis, 1983). They may be frightened by the possible consequences of the condition, without realising fully what they are. Service practitioners need to appreciate these difficulties and offer carers support and advice to enable them to adapt and come to terms with the situation.

To summarise:

- Physical disabilities affect young and older people, and cover a wide range of conditions each having different consequences for the carer.

- Carers of physically disabled people face a physically demanding role which often necessitates intimate care. Many carers experience difficulties with this and service practitioners should not take their involvement for granted.

- Besides undertaking physical and personal care tasks carers also feel a sense of responsibility for the cared-for person.

- The cared-for person's decisions and preferences, although given prominence, do not necessarily reflect those of the carer. Service practitioners need to take both the disabled person's and the carer's wishes into account when making decisions.

Learning disability

Learning disability is a generic term covering a range of disabilities. Most are congenital affecting a child's brain function and learning ability. The causes are varied and sometimes unknown. Common examples include Downs Syndrome, hydrocephalus, and hypercalcaemia. Some forms of learning disability, however, result from more serious forms of brain damage, and entail profound mental and physical disability. These represent about one-third of conditions classified as learning disabilities (Bone and Meltzer, 1991).

The carer's role is obviously affected by the type of learning disability of the cared-for person. Where the cared-for person has a profound mental and physical disability, physical tending remains a central aspect of the carer's role and the literature describes how these carers have to get the cared-for person up in the morning, wash and dress him or her, as well as deal with continence problems (Bayley, 1973; Wilkin, 1979; Tyne, 1982; Ayer and Alaszewski, 1984).

Even those carers who do not have to undertake a heavy burden of physical care can still face difficulties associated with having to assume responsibility for another person. Indeed assuming responsibility for another person is a central feature of the carers' role

(Inechin *et al.*, 1980; Quine and Pahl, 1985; Jones, 1988; Twigg and Atkin, 1993). Such carers may be reluctant to leave the cared-for person alone because they are anxious about what might happen in their absence. Carers often feel answerable for the cared-for person and responsible for future decisions about their life. These carers can also face difficulties as a consequence of sharing their lives with someone who has a disability. Carers of people with learning disabilities identify as particular problems difficult behaviour, such as uncooperative and demanding behaviour, the possibility of self injury, the need for constant attention and insistent talking (Bayley, 1973; Carr, 1976; Jaehnig, 1979; Byrne and Cunningham, 1985; Hubert, 1990). On a daily basis carers find this extremely stressful. The problems that result from assuming responsibility for another person and sharing your life with a disabled person are often difficult to articulate (Twigg and Atkin, 1993) and do not have the same 'objective' quality as physical tasks. As a result, their consequences are sometimes missed by service providers.

As we have noted, many parental carers feel guilty and blame themselves for their child's disability (Chetwynd, 1985; Byrne and Cunningham, 1985; Quine and Pahl, 1985; Clarkson *et al.*, 1986). Mothers, for example, often feel they have done something wrong during pregnancy. Information on the origins of the condition can, therefore, be of considerable importance to the carer. Carers also have to come to terms with the initial shock and sometimes dismay of having a child with a learning disability. The initial period after the birth can be extremely difficult for the family as they try to come to terms with the situation. Carers, for example, may be frightened by the possible consequences of the condition and how they are going to cope with it.

Securing an acceptable future provision after their death is also a worry for many of these carers (Jones, 1988; Ritchie and Richardson, 1989; Twigg and Atkin, 1993). Particular anxieties about future provision include the type of caring arrangements that will be offered to their child as well as concerns about financial provision. Carers often have views on future provision and may favour certain types of accommodation, such as small hostels with a permanent care worker attached, which offer them greater peace of mind.

Turning now to the involvement of service delivery, particular ideas and philosophies such as normalisation and independent living inform the provision of services for people with learning difficulties, and this has importance consequences for how the relationship between the carer and cared-for person is seen (Allen *et al.*, 1990; Ward, 1990). Carers often expect to exercise considerable power over decisions regarding the cared-for person's life. Service practitioners, however, have begun to question this and carers' views, although respected, are no longer given primacy (Further

43

Education Unit, 1990; Hurbert, 1990; McGrath and Grant, 1992; Twigg and Atkin, 1992). As a result, carers can feel that their needs are overlooked by service providers, and they may feel threatened by these changes.

In addition the moves to normalisation and independent living can, from the carers' point of view, reduce the effectiveness of service provision. Moves away from Adult Training Centres to more community-based forms of provision mean that carers can no longer rely on one placement in a recognised building. These changes can increase the carer's anxiety about the whereabouts of the cared-for person (Twigg and Atkin, 1993). Normalisation, although bringing many benefits, can be a source of conflict between carers and service practitioners, as well as creating tensions between the carer and cared-for person. The interests of the carer and cared-for person, therefore, have to be balanced carefully.

To summarise:

- Assuming responsibility for the cared-for person is usually a more important aspect of caring for someone with a learning disability than the performance of physical care tasks, except when the cared-for person has a profound learning and physical disability.

- Normalisation, although bringing many benefits, can cause carers anxiety, as well as creating tensions between them and the cared-for person. Service practitioners, therefore, have to balance carefully the interests of the carer and cared-for person.

Mental health problems

The literature on informal care does not usually include carers of younger people diagnosed as having mental health problems. Traditional views of caring have a strong task orientation and this means that caring for someone with a mental health problem is not regarded as caring (Perring *et al.*, 1990). These carers, although rarely performing physical tending, do have to assume responsibility for the other person, as well as deal with the consequences of sharing their life with them. In these respects, someone looking after a person with mental health problems can be regarded as a carer.

The two features described above lie at the heart of the difficulties that carers face. Assuming responsibility for the life of another person, although common to all caregiving situations, is central in caring for someone with mental health problems (Perring *et al.*, 1990). This can mean providing a home, coping with money or public authorities, managing periodic crises or hospitalization, trying to prevent the cared-for person falling into lethargy and self neglect (Creer *et al.*, 1982). Mental health problems can disrupt family life and impose a social isolation that reinforces guilt and stigma.

Disturbed behaviour, for example, causes great distress and social embarrassment for all family members. The literature describes the reluctance of other members in inviting people to the house (Fadden et al., 1987a; Johnson et al., 1984). Spouse carers find it difficult to maintain a joint social life if one partner is withdrawn and apathetic. In general, carers of people with a mental health problem feel they have to cope with a world that does not want to understand their situation and consequently they feel lonely and trapped (Kreisman and Joy, 1974; Thompson and Doll, 1982; Gibbons et al., 1984). It is not surprising, therefore, that the need to talk about their feelings of loneliness, guilt, and of being stigmatized is of considerable importance to these carers

As with all disabilities, the onset of a mental health problem is a particularly stressful time for the carer during which they may have to come to terms with a fundamental change in a person (Platt, 1985; Creer et al., 1987). Carers may experience an acute sense of loss and bereavement because of this change. Behaviour may have altered to such an extent that carers feel they are living with a completely different person (Perring et al., 1990). In addition carers are often uncertain how to respond. They do not want to be unsympathetic to the person they look after, yet can feel frustrated and baffled by their behaviour (Fadden et al., 1987b; Perring et al., 1990). Carers identify support and reassurance, as well as information and advice about how to cope with onset and with possible future crises as particularly important.

In exploring the consequences of looking after someone with a mental health problem, it is important to remember that there is no single 'mental illness', and different types of mental health problems have different consequences and meanings for the carer. There is an important distinction to be drawn between schizophrenia and psychotic conditions on the one hand and neurotic conditions on the other. Schizophrenia and psychotic conditions are seen more as 'mind disorders', which involve some impairment of cognitive function, particularly in relation to perception and thinking. These conditions can involve difficult behaviour, such as unpredictability, aggression, mood swings, lack of motivation, and withdrawal (Grad and Sainsbury, 1963; Creer and Wing, 1974; Creer, 1975; Vaughn and Leff, 1981; Fadden et al., 1987a). Specific examples include the cared for person shutting him or herself in a room, lacking confidence to seek a social life outside the home, and becoming increasingly demanding of his or her family. Neurotic conditions on the other hand are often characterised by a single predominating symptom, such as feelings of anxiety, depression, and obsessive, compulsive or phobic behaviour. People who are diagnosed as neurotic can show a range of behaviour including threatened or attempted suicide, withdrawn behaviour with no inclination to speak, obsessive behaviour as well as hypochondrial preoccupations.

The difficulties associated with both neurotic and psychotic conditions can be episodic in character. This is true of conditions such as schizophrenia where the sufferer may experience bouts of florid behaviour interspersed with periods of relative stability (Creer and Wing, 1974), as well as conditions such as depression. The variable nature of caring means the carers' needs will change. For example, carers may not require service support for several months, but may need immediate help at the onset of a crisis.

The meaning ascribed to psychotic and neurotic conditions differs. In some respects it is easier to construe schizophrenia and psychotic disorders as 'objective' conditions which have simply occurred. The individual's actions can be attributed to a definite illness state rather than the individual (Perring et al., 1990). Neurotic conditions appear to involve more interpersonal elements (Vaughn and Leff, 1981; Fadden et al., 1987b). There is some evidence to suggest that in the latter case carers respond to anxiety in the cared-for person by showing symptoms of anxiety, whereas carers looking after someone with a psychotic disorder are more likely to adapt to the situation (Fadden et al., 1987a).

The differences in experience and meaning of mental health problems are strongly mediated by the relationship of the carer to the cared-for person. Schizophrenia usually manifests itself in the teens or twenties when the cared-for person is about to establish an independent adult life. Their carers are usually parents who are often concerned about the future (Goldman, 1980). Older carers in particular are anxious about the continuation of suitable care once they themselves are unable to offer support (Perring et al., 1990). Spouse carers on the other hand are more likely to care for people who suffer from conditions such as depression. These carers are less concerned about the future but more distressed by the changes in their marital role (Perring et al., 1990). In this respect spouse carers find withdrawal and apathy particularly difficult to deal with.

Looking after someone with mental health problems, as we have seen, although different from other forms of disability, raises particular difficulties for carers. Their experience, however, is less likely to be recognised by mental health service provision (Perring et al., 1990). First, carers usually have contact with a service characterised by a predominant medical focus which emphasises the individual patient and the medical aspects of their need (Kuipers, 1979, 1987; Fallon et al., 1982). Secondly, the concern of these services is to encourage the independence of the person diagnosed as mentally ill rather than to endorse their dependence on another person. Ideas such as respite, which provides both day-time and more long-term relief, for example, are rarely considered. Where a placement at a day hospital is offered the concern is usually with its therapeutic value to the cared-for person rather than with any benefits that the carer might receive.

Carers, however, would benefit from service support. The need to talk to someone about their feelings, being reassured, as well as obtaining advice and information on how to cope with a family member who is diagnosed as mentally ill are of considerable importance to the carer. Carers in this situation would find contact with service practitioners useful. Carers, however, identify poor long-term involvement with professional workers as a particular problem and they often have difficulties contacting a practitioner especially at times of crisis.

To summarise:

- Mental illness is not a homogeneous category and service practitioners need to understand the consequence for carers of different types of mental health problems.

- The consequences of sharing your life with someone with a mental health problem and being responsible for that person are more significant aspects of the carer's experience than physical tending.

- The experience of carers is rarely recognised in mental health services, which focus predominantly on the needs of the cared-for person. Practitioners need to recognise the role of the carer and how caring for someone with a mental health problem affects their lives.

Older people

Although not all older people are in need of care, it is true that the incidence and severity of disability increase with age. Consequently a growing number of older people implies a growing population of people who need care (Parker, 1990). It is, however, important to remember that older people may need support because they are disabled and not because they are old. With this is mind there are two particular aspects of disability that will be covered in this section – physical disability and mental infirmity.

Physical disability
Caring for an older person with a physical disability is similar to caring for a younger physically disabled person. Physical care tasks and personal tending, for example, are likely to be central to the carer's experience (see above). Older people with a physical disability, therefore, often need help with bathing, dressing, getting in and out of bed, lifting, toileting, as well as with household activities

(Bowling, 1984; Wright, 1986; Levin *et al.*, 1989; Hunter *et al.*, 1988; Lewis and Meredith, 1988; Sinclair, 1990). Not surprisingly carers face a physically demanding role and this creates particular problems if the carer is old and in poor health, as is often the case amongst carers of older people with a physical disability. Only a third of carers of older people say their own health is good, and about half have disabilities themselves (Green, 1988; Levin *et al.*, 1989). Consequently support with physical care tasks, in which services substitute for the carer, are much valued by the carer.

There are difficulties specific to older carers concerning the onset of disability. Relatives of older people tend to become carers gradually as the level of disability increases. These carers drift, often without realising it, into offering support and help; in some cases the carer might see it as a natural extension of their family role without seeing themselves as a carer (Ungerson, 1983; Lewis and Meredith, 1988). Consequently many of these carers remain unknown to service practitioners, and the carers' needs are often acted upon only in the event of a crisis. In other cases, such as strokes, onset can be sudden with little or no warning. Onset of disability in these circumstances means that the carer's life becomes transformed overnight.

To summarise:

- Carers of older people face a physically demanding role and this creates particular problems if the carer is also old and in poor health.

- Relatives of older people tend to become carers gradually, often without realising it. Consequently many of these carers remain unknown to service practitioners, and their needs are often acted upon only in the event of a crisis.

Mental infirmity
Looking after an older person with a mental infirmity is identified as being particularly stressful for a carer. Mental infirmity destroys the ability to remember, think and reason. It strikes at the very core of a person's being and is often described in the literature as 'tragic', 'daunting' and 'destructive' (Lewis and Meredith, 1988; Levin *et al.*, 1989).

Carers who live with someone with a mental infirmity face a whole series of behavioural and interpersonal problems including the inability of the cared-for person to converse normally, restlessness, unsafe acts such as forgetting to turn off the gas, wandering, not recognising the carer, hitting out at the carer, and disturbing the carer's sleep (Gilhooly, 1982; Gilleard *et al.*, 1984; Smith and Cantley, 1985; Wright, 1986; Lewis and Meredith, 1988; Levin *et al.*, 1989). In addition to these, the carer may also have to deal with physical problems resulting from conditions such as arthritis and rheumatism and chronic bronchitis, as well as incontinence (Levin et al., 1989; Sinclair, 1990). Since the older person is also regarded as being incapable of making decisions about and organising their own life, the carer has to assume responsibility for the cared-for person (Lewis and Meredith, 1988; Levin et al., 1989).

Changes in personality and behavioural difficulties can be particularly distressing (Gilhooly, 1982; Gilleard et al., 1984; Lewis and Meredith, 1988; Levin et al., 1989). Carers may experience an acute sense of loss and bereavement and feel that they are living with someone completely different. In this respect mental infirmity erodes the relationship between carer and the cared-for person. The cared-for person, for example, often does not even recognise the person who looks after him or her, and this is especially painful for carers. Not surprisingly carers experience a range of emotions which include feelings of guilt, pity, impatience, repugnance, and embarrassment, as well as great love and affection (Lewis and Meredith, 1988; Levin et al., 1989; Sinclair, 1990; Hills, 1991).

Caring can also have an enormous impact on other aspects of the carer's life. Carers are often prevented from getting out and meeting family and friends because of the cared-for person's need for constant support, supervision and attention (Lewis and Meredith, 1988; Levin et al., 1989; Sinclair, 1990). Caring can also impose considerable strain on the carer's material resources (Gilleard et al., 1982; Wright, 1986; Gilhooly, 1986; Lewis and Meredith, 1988). If carers are under retirement age caring can affect their ability to go to work. The cared-for person's infirmity may have other financial implications including extra expenditure on keeping the house warm, for laundry, and for replacing clothing and furnishings.

The difficulties experienced by these carers, and the impact of caring on their lives are extremely stressful. Indeed, evidence suggests that despite the carers' willingness to care, they are generally worn down, over time, by the strain of caring. It is reported, for example, that the greatest improvement in the mental health of carers of older people with a mental infirmity came with the death or institutionalisation of the person they looked after (Levin et al., 1989). This is not to say that these carers would necessarily have wished for such an outcome, but it is important to understand that many carers continue to give care, despite finding it extremely difficult to do so.

Service practitioners, therefore, have an important responsibility to these carers. A carer may not find individual tasks difficult but can be overwhelmed by the whole caring situation (Levin et al., 1989). Evidence suggests various forms of intervention are useful. For example, due to the need to offer continued support and supervision carers need regular periods of respite (Levin et al., 1989;

Sinclair, 1990). Another key requirement for services is that they make early identification of the carer's problems (Levin *et al.*, 1989; Sinclair, 1990; Hills, 1991). This enables service practitioners to reduce the carer's stress at an early stage rather than when the carer is exhausted. Furthermore, because confusion is a condition that deteriorates progressively, there is a need for continuing medical and social assessments as well as back-up support. Continuous rather than one-off support is required (Levin *et al.*, 1989; Sinclair, 1990).

Providing information, advice and counselling is also identified by carers as important (Gilhooly, 1984; Levin *et al.*, 1989; Sinclair, 1990; Hills, 1991). Particular shortfalls identified by carers include difficulties in finding out about the cared-for person's condition and obtaining advice on how to cope with behavioural difficulties. Often carers do not know what to do for the best and are baffled by bizarre behaviour. Carers often need emotional support as they come to terms with sadness and loneliness, as well as anger, resentment and frustration. They have, however, no recognised point of contact that enables them to receive this sort of information and support, and rarely receive systematic advice.

To summarise:

- Carers of older people with dementia face a series of behavioural, interpersonal and social problems, as well as the possibility of physical tending and incontinence.

- Despite carers' willingness to care, over time they are generally worn down by the strain of caring. Early and continuous intervention is, therefore, necessary.

- Providing information, advice and counselling is identified as particularly important by carers. In addition, due to the need for continued support and supervision, carers need regular breaks, as well as help in relieving the more general difficulties of caring.

The carer's background

In the previous sections we explored the differences that arise as a result of the relationship of the carer and cared-for person and the disability of the cared-for person. This section explores more structural aspects of the carer's situation relating to factors such as gender, age, social class, race and geographical location.

Gender

The issue of gender has always been at the centre of the debate on informal care (Finch and Groves, 1983; Ungerson, 1983, 1987; Land

and Rose, 1985). Indeed the issue of informal care was first brought on to the policy agenda by feminists wishing to analyse the unequal burdens being imposed on women and to reclaim the ways in which women's home activities constituted work. From this a critique of community care policy developed in which informal care was seen as oppressive to women.

As we have seen in the previous chapter, recent work, although highlighting the large number of male carers, still points to gender differences in the provision of care. Women are more likely to become carers than men, and where caring for somebody other than a spouse, more likely to be providing personal care. Caring is still regarded by both carers and service providers as intimately related to the female role and to domestic labour. Women are often depicted as 'natural carers', and better able to cope with the demands of care-giving than men (Gilligan, 1982; Dalley, 1987; Ungerson, 1987; Lewis and Meredith, 1988). Indeed certain tasks are seen as more suitable for women to carry out than men (Ungerson, 1982; Lewis and Meredith, 1988). For example, personal care is, by definition, inti-mate in nature, often involving touching, nakedness and contact with excreta (Twigg, 1990). The different cultural treatment of men's and women's bodies in relation to bodily contact may mean that a man's role is more highly constrained than a woman's. Consequently the intimate labour of personal care is more associ-ated with women than men, and men who undertake these tasks are more likely to be regarded as needing support (Ungerson, 1987). Household tasks raise similar issues. Twigg and Atkin (1993) report a home care organiser as saying that she would automatically estab-lish home help support to a working man, but would have to think about it for a working woman. These assumptions have important implications for the visibility of female carers and the support they receive. The domestic role of a woman, for example, often obscures her caring role; a man undertaking similar tasks is more likely to be identified as a carer because his support is regarded as in some way extraordinary.

These gendered assumptions are often held as much by the carers as by the service providers, and this can affect what help is regarded as appropriate (Lewis and Meredith, 1988; Twigg and Atkin, 1993). A different personal meaning is ascribed to certain caring tasks, and this can play a part in the seeking of support and in its acceptance when it is offered. Women, for example, are less like-ly to perceive help with household tasks as appropriate; and men appear to find it easier and more natural to accept help in these areas. Service practitioners, therefore, have to be able to distinguish between what the carer really needs and what the carer feels he or she can ask for. Careful negotiation is often required.

To summarise:

- The issue of gender has always been at the centre of the informal care debate. From this a critique of community care policy developed in which informal care was seen as oppressive to women.

- Gendered assumptions are evident in the responses of service practitioners and these can disadvantage female carers. Men are not only likely to be more visible to service practitioners, but also more likely to be seen as needing support.

- Gendered assumptions are reflected not only in the service practitioners' priorities but also that of the carer. Service practitioners, therefore, have to be able to distinguish between what the carer really needs and what the carer feels he or she can ask for.

Age

Society is to a large degree structured by age. A person's age has important implications for how he or she is seen by others, as well as for the social-economic resources he or she commands. This can have important ramifications for informal care.

In general most older people endure poorer social conditions than the rest of the population. The patterns of disadvantage they face, such as bad housing, poverty and low income as well as social isolation, low social status and relative lack of power are well documented (Walker, 1980; Norman, 1980; Townsend, 1981; Phillipson, 1982; Fennell et al., 1989; Parker, 1990). Perhaps not surprisingly there is usually a great difference in the socio-economic resources available to young and older carers. People with resources can buy help, adapt their homes, use taxis and employ other means to ensure their continued participation in social life. They can also, of course, buy care. However, with 50 per cent of older people living in poverty, such options are likely only to be available to younger carers (Townsend, 1982; Arber and Ginn, 1991). Moreover, older people experience greater social isolation than younger people. Even in rural communities one in twenty older people report that they never receive a visit from a close relative. This figure is much higher in urban areas – in Greater London only one quarter received a visit from a relative more than once a week and one in six never received a visit (Sinclair et al., 1990).

Age can also have an impact on informal care in more direct ways. First, a significant proportion of older carers report some form of physical disability. This can often add to the difficulties of their caring role, particularly if the cared-for person requires physical tending; lifting and manoeuvring a disabled person has been identified as causing particular problems (Lewis and Meredith, 1988; Levin et al., 1989). Moreover in some spouse relationships, where both husband and wife experience poor health or disability, older people can be seen to be caring for each other (Sinclair, 1990). Younger carers, by comparison, are less likely to be in poor health. Secondly, for an older person caring for someone younger, the primary concern is with the future and what will happen after their death to the person they look after. The concerns of younger carers, however, are different. Worries about the future, although common, do not assume the same degree of urgency (Twigg and Atkin, 1993).

Older carers can also face disadvantage in their contact with service practitioners. Interventions by service practitioners are often guided by the age of the carer and informed by an idea of what normal life is like for different age groups. Although younger carers are seen as needing less support with physical tasks than older carers, older carers are seen as less likely to need a social life. Evidence from Twigg and Atkin's study suggests that developing a social life for a younger carer was seen as a legitimate use of social work resources; social workers, however, were less concerned to provide this sort of help when the carer was older (Twigg and Atkin, 1993). Generalised cultural expectations are, however, not an adequate basis on which to offer support; some older carers may require help in maintaining a social life. Service practitioners, therefore, need to respond according to the needs of each situation rather than on cultural expectations of age.

To summarise:

- Age has important implications for a person's socio-economic and political resources, with most older people enduring poorer social conditions than the rest of the population. This affects the options available to them.

- Older carers are more likely to be in poor health than younger carers and therefore experience greater difficulty with physical care tasks. Older carers are also more likely to have more immediate concerns about the future of the person they look after.

- Service practitioners' interventions are often informed by an idea of what normal life is like for different age groups. Service practitioners, however, need to respond according to the needs of each situation rather than on cultural expectations of age.

Race and ethnicity
With an estimated 2.57 million people from black and ethnic minorities living in this country, representing about five per cent of the total population, Britain is a multi-racial society. As we have seen in Chapter One demography exerts powerful influences on policy formulation, and it represents a useful starting point in discussing the policy debate on social care and race (Atkin and Rollings, 1992).

First, black and ethnic minority populations are not an homogeneous group. South Asian (Indian, Pakistani and Bangladeshi) people comprise over half the total minority population, while Afro/Caribbean people make up just over a quarter of the total population (Shaw, 1988). Other minority groups who have settled in Britain include African, Chinese, Arab, Jewish and Polish people. Policy needs to reflect this diversity. Secondly, the uneven geographical distribution of black and minority ethnic communities presents local agencies with a variety of challenges in meeting service needs.The highest populations of people from black and ethnic minorities occur generally in London and the metropolitan counties, and the lowest in non-metropolitan counties, particularly those in the south west, the north and Wales (OPCS, 1984). Thirdly, the relationship between age and disability indicates the importance of the age distribution of black and ethnic minority communities. Minority groups are, on average, younger than white populations. Whereas a fifth of all private household residents in Great Britain are aged 60 and over, this is the case for only four per cent of South East Asian and six per cent of Afro/Caribbean people. Demographic trends, however, indicate an imminent growth in the numbers of older people of Afro/Caribbean and Asian descent (Williams, 1990). The rising proportion of older people (that is, those aged between 45-60) among Afro/Caribbean people (19 per cent) and Asian people (12 per cent), for example, is comparable to that of white people (19 per cent). Fourthly, differences in the numbers of men and women affect the populations of those who need care, and of those who take on the responsibility of care (Fenton, 1987). Men from black and ethnic minorities will outnumber women for a decade or so despite greater female longevity.

There is little work on informal care among black and ethnic minorities. Yet being black is an important aspect of a person's experience (Kiple and King, 1981; Norman, 1985; Donovan, 1987; Cameron et al., 1989), and the disadvantage black people face in health, education, housing, and employment is well documented (Rex and Mason, 1986; Carr-Hill and Harbajan Chadha-Boreham, 1988; NAHA, 1988; Bandana Ahmad, 1989). Racism is agreed to be central to understanding this disadvantage. Black people do not have the same opportunities as white people because of discrimination against them on the grounds of having a different skin colour. Black people's lifestyles, for example, are seen as different from those of the white population and this difference becomes seen as something deviant or pathological. The idea that black people have 'special needs' can be an example of this (Atkin, 1991a).

The unsuitability and inaccessible nature of community service provision to people who form black and ethnic minorities is equally well established, with many authors arguing that services are ethnocentric and grounded in racist assumptions (Hughes, 1986; Prime, 1987; Hughes and Bhaduri, 1987; Cypher, 1988; Dominelli, 1989; Evers *et al.*, 1989; Whitfield, 1990; Atkin, 1991b). Service provision is often organised around a white norm. A day centre might only provide English food, which ignores the preferences of black clients. Rules and regulations that apply to all can have an effect of excluding black people while maintaining the privileged position of white people. For example waiting lists for local authority housing which exclude people who have not lived in an area for a certain number of years discriminate against black people. There is also the problem of unchallenged stereotypes and myths among service practitioners (Hughes and Bhaduri, 1987; Pearson, 1988).

In relation to informal care the idea that black people 'look after their own' is perhaps the most common. The commitment of black families to care for older and disabled relatives is assumed to be greater than that of white people, to the extent that service provision thinks it need not concern itself with the needs of black people. Research into the circumstances of black family networks, however, draws attention to that fact that the supportive extended family is largely a myth (Fenton, 1987; Baxter, 1989; Atkin, 1992). A third of Afro/Caribbean older people, for example, live alone and the number who live in three generational households is similar to that of white people. Although the extended family is common among Asian families, there is still a significant proportion who live alone, with few relatives in this country. The traditional pattern in many Asian communities of the responsibility of care being shared among a network of family members is not so readily achievable in Great Britain. First, migrant families are often divided by migration itself, and this is further exacerbated by post-1962 legislation and administration of immigration policy. Secondly, changes in family and household structure as well as the geographical dispersal of kin make it increasingly difficult for Asian family life to continue around the extended kinship network. In any case living within a large family does not necessarily mean that service support is not needed; a recent study, for example, suggested that an expressed need for respite service was twice as high for Asian families as for white families (Robinson and Stalker, 1992).

To summarise:

- Britain is a multi-racial society and this cannot be ignored by service practitioners.

- The disadvantage black people face in health, education, housing and employment is well documented. Racism is central to understanding this disadvantage.

- Racism is also fundamental in understanding how service practitioners respond to black people. The unsuitability and inaccessible nature of community service provision to people who form black and ethnic minorities is well established.

Social class

The incidence of informal care is not related to social class; working-class people are not more likely to care than middle-class people (Green, 1988). Co-resident care, however, which places greater constraints on the carer's life, is more frequently provided by working-class than middle-class men and women, and Arber and Ginn therefore argue that working-class people bear the 'greatest burden' of care (Arber and Ginn, forthcoming).

Social class has important consequences for a person's socio-economic as well as political resources. As such it provides an important background to the context of caring and is significant in determining the options available to different families.

First, middle-class carers usually have access to greater material resources than working-class carers. Evidence from America on families who have a member diagnosed as mentally ill suggests that middle-class families are more likely to use money and resources while working-class families are more likely to use time, goods and physical space (Gubman and Tessler, 1987). Middle-class carers, in particular, might have extra money to increase their caring options, perhaps buying in care (Parker, 1990). Old people in social classes I and II, for example, are not only more likely to use a private nursing or old people's home than a local authority facility (Townsend, 1962; Sinclair, 1990b) but also enter nursing homes at a more advanced age or when more frail than their working-class counterparts (Wade, et al., 1983). In general higher incomes and higher social class are associated with the avoidance of admission to residential care among older people in the community (Wenger, 1984).

Secondly, caring has a differential impact on labour market participation between manual workers and non-manual workers – people with manual jobs are more likely to have to give up their jobs to care (Parker, 1990). Indeed the largest differences in labour market participation between fathers of severely disabled children and fathers of non-disabled children occurred among unskilled manual workers; their participation rates being 76.2 percent and 90 per cent respectively (Baldwin, 1985).

Social class is also an important variable in considering the response of service practitioners (Friedson, 1970; Arber and Ginn, 1991). First, middle-class people are more likely to know about the availability of service provision. A recent study of respite services, for example, illustrates that families where the father had a semi-skilled occupation were less likely to know about respite services than families where the father had a skilled or non-manual occupation (Robinson and Stalker, 1992). Secondly, middle-class social skills and powers of articulation seem to make it more likely that they are known to service practitioners than their working-class counterparts (Ungerson, 1987; Buckquet and Curtis, 1986; Rojek et al., 1988). Middle-class people, for example, tend to have more productive consultations with general practitioners partly because they see them as having a wider social role. The general practitioner is regarded as a powerful ally, as well as a resource enabling access to other services. Working-class people, on the other hand, are more likely to define the work of the general practitioner in narrow medical terms (Stimson and Webb, 1975; Cartwright and O'Brien, 1976). The contact that middle- and working-class clients have with social workers seems to follow a similar pattern (Mayer and Timms, 1970; Robinson, 1978). Middle-class clients are more likely to be pro-active in their dealing with social workers, seeing them as a stepping stone to other services, whereas working-class clients are more likely to be passive and accepting about what is offered to them (Meethan, 1990).

To summarise:

- Social class has important consequences for a person's socio-economic, as well as political resources. Middle-class carers usually have access to better material resources than working-class carers. Middle-class carers are also more likely to have jobs that offer greater flexibility in which to accommodate their caring role.

- Social class is also an important variable in considering the response of service practitioners. Working-class people are often disadvantaged in their contacts with service practitioners.

Geographical differences
The importance of geographical variations in the delivery of services has been well established in the literature (Agnew, 1987; Bagguley et al., 1990; Cook, 1990; Harloe et al., 1990). The implications of this for informal care are twofold.

First, service delivery is subject to political decision making, and different authorities have different priorities (Davies, Day and Klein, 1987; Harloe et al., 1990; Meethan, 1990). It is therefore not surprising that the pattern of service delivery varies between geographical regions. For carers with similar needs the support available to them will vary according to locality.

Secondly, social, economic, gender, ethnic and class differences can combine in various ways to constitute a locality that has particular social care needs (Wenger, 1984; Meethan and Thompson, 1991). In some areas, for example, older people, because of changing family structure, may find it difficult to obtain the support of kin (Finch, 1991). This is particularly true in some coastal areas, where older people may have migrated many miles from other family members; or in economically depressed areas, where younger family members have moved away to find work (Sinclair, 1990).

Urban and rural areas present different problems for service delivery (Wenger, 1984; Osmond, 1992). According to the myth of rural life, rural communities are relatively wealthy and local problems are solved through self help (Bagguley *et al.*, 1990). Although there is no evidence to support this it is often used to justify the lack of service support in rural communities, but carers living in rural areas are just as likely to require support as carers living in urban areas (Harloe *et al.*, 1990). Organising support in rural areas is difficult because of the dispersed population. The costs of service delivery, therefore, are likely to be higher in rural areas because of this. Rural dispersal also creates difficulties in bringing together people with specific difficulties. Organising a day centre that is accessible to all people can become a problem. Overall, carers living in rural areas are likely to face greater difficulties than those living in urban areas.

To summarise:

- Patterns of service delivery vary between geographical regions and carers with similar needs will often find the support available to them different according to the locality in which they live.

- Social, economic, gender, ethnic and class differences can combine in various ways to constitute a locality that has particular social care needs.

3

Carers in the service system

JULIA TWIGG

The role of mainstream services

In the final two chapters of this review, we examine the role of different services in the support of carers. In this chapter we concentrate on 'mainstream' services; and in Chapter Four on innovations and special projects and some of the management issues they raise. It is not always easy to distinguish between mainstream services and innovative ones. This is partly because 'innovation' often takes place within mainstream services, altering the way a service is provided or the philosophy of care that underlies it, and to this degree innovation represents the process of change itself.

The division we adopt here is a pragmatic one. 'Mainstream' services are taken to be those that we can expect to find in all or most localities. They are usually provided in the statutory sector, and are often governed by legislation. They cover the familiar range of health and social services; and they are often provided as much for the cared-for person as for the carer.

'Innovations' and special projects, by contrast, are specialist forms of support that are not found everywhere. They depend for their existence on a specific and often one-off decision to provide them. They cannot be assumed to be available. They tend to have a limited geographical scope, which means that their coverage is patchy. Carers often complain that the innovative services they read about in handbooks do not exist in their locality. Systematic attempts to map availability endorse this picture of uneven provision (Moore and Green, 1985; Twigg, 1988). Such services are often – though not necessarily – provided in the voluntary sector, and suffer from the instability of funding characteristic of that sector. They are frequently small in scale, and as a result have a limited ability to take on new cases. Although we term them 'innovative', many have been around in service thinking for some time; for example, flexible

59

forms of home-based respite have been available in some areas for the last two decades. What continues to mark them as 'innovations' is their failure to establish themselves as standard forms of service.

Although it is hard to quantify the level of inputs from various service sectors, studies that look across the range of services tend to conclude that it is mainstream services that provide the bulk of help that currently goes to carers (Levin *et al.*, 1989; Twigg and Atkin, 1993). This is not to say that innovative services are unimportant. They have a particularly vital role to play in altering the assumptions of planners and practitioners about what can or should be provided. Their scope is, however, limited. The bulk of support that currently comes to carers does so from mainstream services.

To summarise:

- 'Mainstream' services are those that are provided in all or most localities; whereas 'innovations' and special schemes are confined to particular places only. The process of innovation is not, however, confined to these special schemes but takes place in mainstream services also.

- Mainstream services are usually found in the statutory sector, and they are often provided for the cared-for person as much as the carer.

- Such services represent the main source of support to carers.

What counts as a service for carers?

One of the problems facing planners in this field is defining what 'counts' as a service for carers. Carers occupy an ambiguous position within the field of social care (Twigg, 1989a). They are not clients or patients, and they are rarely the main focus of service provision. As we have noted, the majority of help that comes to them does so from services aimed primarily at the person they look after. Because of the close interrelationship between the carer and the cared-for person, there is a sense in which *all* help to the cared-for person is relevant to the carer also. This does not mean that there are no potential conflicts of interest between the two, and we shall explore further some of the implications of these below; it does however mean that what 'counts' as a service needs to be envisaged widely.

It is helpful to think of services for carers as existing in three forms:

Specific carer services. These are services that are unambiguously provided to carers. They often have the word carer or relative in the title. Carer support groups, or the Crossroads Care Attendant Schemes provide classic examples. They tend to be small in scale and are often found in the voluntary sector. Some mainstream services such as respite are also included in this category. These services are traditionally perceived as central in the support of carers.

Carer allocations. Carers also receive help from mainstream services aimed primarily at the person they look after. Sometimes the allocation is explicit, as for example when a day care place is provided for the cared-for person with the intention of relieving the carer. Sometimes it happens less overtly, as a by- product of assistance to the cared-for person. Such allocations can be very important in supporting carers, but they are hard to trace in a service system geared to the support of clients and patients.

Service assumptions and practices. Beyond these specific services and allocations, there is a more global level. Service providers make assumptions about carers – their availability, their duties, their likely involvement – and to some degree structure their provision in the light of them. These embedded assumptions and practices can have major implications for carers, for example through their impact on the way the ambulance service is organised, or the assumptions that the consultant makes at point of discharge about the 'availability' of relatives. They are not 'carer services' as such, but represent the way in which the system as a whole has an impact on the lives of carers.

To summarise:
- Services for carers should not be confined to the specific carer services but need to encompass the way the service system *as a whole* relates to and has an impact on the situation of carers.

- All three forms of 'service' need to be addressed if the needs of carers are to be met and the service system made more carer sensitive.

What are the relevant service sectors?

It is sometimes assumed that caring is a social-services issue, with some involvement by the voluntary sector. Certainly in the past the bulk of specific services for carers was found in these sectors, where general awareness of the issue was also more developed. Health services, by contrast, have not traditionally perceived carers as an issue central to their concerns and responsibilities. This has been particularly true of the acute sector, whose interests traditionally dominate the health service. Perceptions are however changing.

Health authorities are increasingly recognising the importance of support for carers; and there have been a number of initiatives – notably the Yorkshire Regional Health Authority Carers' Project – that have attempted to promote the needs of carers among the concerns of health authorities.

Of course, health services, particularly those that are community based, have always been significant for carers. Many carers are in touch *only* with health services, and the degree to which their needs are recognised and met often depends on the sensitivity and awareness of medical and nursing staff. Furthermore, many services, such as respite, are provided by all three service sectors: health, social services and the voluntary sector.

To summarise:
- Issues concerning carers transcend the boundaries of health and social care.

- All three service sectors – health, social services and voluntary – need to consider the issue and be aware of the impact of their responses.

Carers as users

The last decade has seen an increasing emphasis on the needs of carers. A large and international literature has explored the difficulties and stresses carers face. The fact that caring is something that large numbers of people do is increasingly appreciated; and the degree to which community care is carried by the work of these informal carers is now well understood. This growing concern was in part fuelled by the feminist critique that emphasised the exploitative character of community care and that exposed the 'compulsory altruism' that underlay it (Wilson, 1982; Finch and Groves, 1983; Graham, 1983, 1991; Land and Rose, 1985; Ungerson, 1987; Dalley, 1988). As a result, the needs of carers are increasingly featured on the policy agenda: politicians express concern about their situation; agencies attempt to support them through services; and in all this, the carer is seen as a legitimate focus for concern and support.

More recently this assumption has been challenged. The growing emphasis on the needs of carers has been criticised within the disability lobby (Oliver, 1990; Morris, 1991). Disabled people are asserting their rights to independence. Channelling support to carers, they argue, simply underwrites dependence. It locks disabled people into relationships of obligation that they want to transcend, diverting money and support from its proper focus which is that of supporting the autonomy and independence of the disabled person. In this view, carers should never be regarded as users.

The critique has itself been criticised for emphasising too much the interests of younger physically disabled people, for whom the aims of autonomy and independence can more easily be endorsed. It is harder to apply these principles to the situation of elderly couples or to conditions like dementia, where it may not be appropriate to think of transcending the caring relationship. These differences underline yet again the importance of recognising that carers are not a homogeneous group. Caring, however, often takes place in a relationship that is characterised by obligation and usually love. In these situations, we need to recognise that carers also have interests. Caring has consequences for their lives, and carers may have service needs that arise from that fact. By this token therefore, carers can legitimately be regarded as users.

To summarise:

- The growing emphasis on the needs of carers does raise issues in relation to disabled people. There is a danger that their needs will be neglected and resources diverted away from their support.

- Autonomy and independence are appropriate expectations for disabled people. But these need to be seen in the context of the obligations that carers can feel. Caring takes place in a relationship.

- There are potential conflicts of interest between the carer and the cared-for person. These need, however, to be interpreted in the context of a relationship which is characterised by obligation, long-term reciprocity and, in most cases, love.

What is the proper relationship between agencies and carers?

As we have seen in relation to the debate on carers as users, carers occupy an ambiguous position within the social care system. This makes it hard to determine the *proper* relationship between them and public agencies. They are not clients or patients, and yet they are part of the concern of welfare agencies. They are rarely the direct focus of an intervention, but service interventions can have major consequences for their lives. Agencies are unsure how far they should be concerned with their well-being *per se*, as opposed to a more instrumental emphasis on ensuring the continuance of their involvement in order to support a disabled client.

Twigg (1989a, 1992) has conceptualised these ambiguities in terms of four models of how public agencies should relate to carers: carers as resources, as co-workers, as co-clients, and superseded carers. Agencies do not hold to any one exclusively, but shift between the different frames of reference according to the particular circumstances that present themselves. Sometimes one will be more appropriate than another.

Carers as resources. This represents the predominant reality of community care: most of the help that comes to disabled and elderly people does so from the informal sector. Informal care represents the taken-for-granted reality against which agencies operate. Informal care is regarded as coming first, with the assumption that services need only step in when it is unavailable. Carers are here regarded as a form of 'resource'. The central focus is on the cared-for person, who is the client. Carers feature only as part of the background, and the agency is largely unconcerned with their welfare. The potential conflict of interest between carer and cared-for person is ignored. The predominant concern is with maximising care; and there is often a fear that the formal services will substitute for informal care.

Carers as co-workers. Here the aim is to work alongside the informal sector, interweaving agency support with that of the carer. Carers are seen as co-workers in a joint care enterprise. The primary focus is still on the client, but in a way that recognises the importance of the morale of the carer, both for the continuance of care and for its quality. The co-worker model thus encompasses the carer's interest and well-being among its concerns, but on an essentially instrumental basis. Conflicts of interest are recognised, but seen as something that can with sensitivity be resolved.

Carers as co-clients. In this model carers are regarded as people in need of help in their own right. Services are aimed at relieving their situation and enhancing their morale. The use of the term 'carer' is however limited, confined only to those cases where the carers are heavily burdened or stressed. The focus of intervention is the carer, and his or her well-being is valued *per se*. The conflict of interest is fully recognised, though the primary emphasis is placed on the problems this poses for the carer.

Superseded carers. Here the aim is not to draw on or support the caregiving relationship, but to transcend or supersede it. There are two different routes to this model. One starts from a concern with the disabled person and maximising his or her independence. The aim is not to ease the lot of carers, but to free disabled people from relationships of dependence with their carers. In some situations the relationship itself is seen as constricting to the disabled persons' growth. The model has been particularly influential in relation to adults with learning disabilities. The second route comes from a concern with the carer. Maximising the independence of the disabled or older person will potentially do away with the need for care and with it the burdens of the carer. Sometimes it is appropriate to think in terms of supporting a carer in the decision to give up care: taking the well-being of carers seriously can mean accepting that only the cessation of caring will result in any significant improvement in morale.

Carers in the superseded model tend not to be to described as such, and the word is replaced by terms like 'relatives' or 'parents' that are more neutral and do not imply the same moral responsibility. The focus of intervention is either on the carer or the disabled person depending on which route has been the influential one. Either way the carer and the cared-for are seen as separate beings. Conflict of interest is fully recognised, and from the viewpoint of both. The valued outcome is independence for both.

To summarise:
- Carers occupy an ambiguous position within the social care system, and agencies have shifting perceptions of their responsibilities to carers.

- Sometimes they emphasis the carer's well-being *per se*. At other times they take a more instrumental – even 'exploitative' – approach.

- Agencies shift between four different models of carers: as resources, as co-clients, as co-workers and as superseded carers.

Mainstream services

We now turn to the principal mainstream services involved in supporting carers. We will start with services organised within social services departments, such as social work and the home care service. We will then explore the role of health services through the work of general practitioners, hospital doctors and the community nursing service. Finally we turn to respite services, and carer support groups – forms of support found in all three service sectors.

Social work

Social workers are the senior and dominant profession in social service departments, and as such they occupy a pivotal position in relation to community care. In the past, casework has been regarded as the core of their work, but increasingly they are seen as the assessors and mobilisers of packages of care. Social workers are important for carers in both these guises.

The training of social workers means that they tend to be more aware of the problems of carers than many other service providers. The clearest contrast is with GPs who occupy a similar pivotal position in relation to the mobilisation of health services, but who tend to be less familiar with carer issues. Of all service providers in Twigg and Atkin's study, social workers were the most aware of the potential conflict of interest between the carer and the cared-for person.

The major stumbling block for carers, however, lies in the fact that few of them come into contact with a trained social worker. Because of the informal specialism that has long existed in social service departments, carers of elderly and disabled people are still largely in contact with untrained staff (Sinclair *et al.*, 1990). More complex cases, however, do get passed to trained social workers, and these often involve family conflict or the transition to institutional care, both of which raise 'carer' issues. Carers of people with learning disabilities are more likely to be in contact with a trained social worker through a specialist learning disability team.

Most social work contact with carers follows the familiar pattern of assessment, referral and case closure found with elderly and disabled clients (Rowlings, 1981). Carers do not always understand this pattern, and sometimes complain when they do not 'have' a social worker as they 'have' a GP. Caring is something that from their perception simply continues over time, and they expect the response of social services to mimic that fact (Twigg and Atkin, 1993). Carers repeatedly praise those practitioners who pop by unasked to talk to them and offer advice. This sort of unfocused visiting is, of course, anathema in professional social work circles (Goldberg and Warburton, 1979). There are a number of reasons why carers value such visits. Caring is isolating, and carers enjoy the chance to talk informally; they often do not perceive this as 'social work'. Carers are unsure of what is available; they want to be told what is possible rather than have to ask. They are often diffident about asking for help for themselves, and need to feel that it is legitimate to do so. A practitioner who comes to them is therefore doubly welcome. Departments, in prioritising their activities, need to consider whether these wishes, if they cannot appropriately be met in this form, can be so in another.

Social workers in the current climate often face problems in relation to carers arising from the limited range of services that they can offer; and Twigg and Atkin found little evidence of social workers going beyond standard services to negotiate complex packages of care. This conclusion is echoed by Allen and her colleagues (1992) in their study of choice and determination in the transition to residential care. They explored the views of carers, elderly people and social workers, but found little evidence of choice or of complex packages of care. The section on the integration of services below discusses this issue further.

To summarise:

- Social workers are well placed to recognise and act upon the needs of carers. Few carers, however, come into contact with a trained social worker.

- Carers value social workers – as they do general practitioners – who call at the house unasked. Such unfocused visits are however counter to dominant models of good practice.

- There is little evidence of social workers – or other practitioners – mobilising complex packages of support for carers.

The home care service

Support to carers has not historically been included among the aims of the home care – formerly home help – service. The way in which the service has traditionally been targeted means that it is effectively biased away from giving such help. Provision is commonly focused on those who live alone and are perceived to be 'unsupported'. These principles largely preclude its use in support of carers. Elderly couples do receive support, but in these cases the service regards both as clients, rather than as client and carer.

The bias towards those who live alone means that the service is systematically targeted away from certain situations that are known to be extremely stressful for carers, and where many would value support. Living with someone who has dementia is a prime example of this. Levin and her colleagues in their study (1989) of the supporters of people with senile dementia found that those carers who were dealing with faecal incontinence, disturbed behaviour and who showed the greatest strain were far less likely to receive home help than were the less heavily burdened. This arose largely out of the bias in allocation against those who shared a household, where the carer had to deal with these difficulties on a twenty-four hour basis. As we shall see, where home help was provided it did alleviate the situation.

Targeting on people who are perceived to be 'unsupported' also has consequences for carers. Many authorities have in the past operated rules that effectively presume the support of relatives. Thus in certain areas, home helps have not traditionally been provided where there is a relative – particularly a female relative – living within a certain distance of the client. These rules are primarily concerned to prevent any substitution of formal for informal support, and they clearly start from an approach to services that regards carers as a form of 'resource' to be drawn on, rather than as people who may need relief in themselves.

There is clear evidence of the helpfulness of the home care service (Sinclair *et al.*, 1990). It is highly valued by its clients; and this positive estimation is found also among carers who receive its support (Levin *et al.*, 1989; Twigg and Atkin, 1993). Home helps are often praised by carers for the practical help that they give. They are also valued for their company and for emotional support. This is particularly important where the carers are themselves elderly and looking after someone with dementia with whom they can no longer have a normal conversation. Visits from the home help can also allow the carer to have a break and to get out of the house for a brief period.

Levin and her colleagues found that receipt of home help could improve the mental health of carers looking after someone with dementia. In the case of male carers, it also appeared to help delay institutionalisation. They speculate on the reasons for this, and suggest that it may result from the 'different personal meaning' of receipt of the service for men and women (Levin *et al.*, 1985). For women, housework is part of their normal expectation and self identity. Other studies have also found women carers more inclined to see housework as either unproblematic or a 'personal matter' – something in relation to which they are not looking for compensatory support in order to make up for the other strains of caring (Ramdas, 1986; Parker, 1992; Twigg and Atkin, 1993).

There is some evidence that the home help service has traditionally been allocated in gender-biased way, though the extent is disputed (Davies and Bebbington, 1983; Arber *et al.*, 1988). In relation to carers, as important as the sex of the carer is is her marital status, with a married woman sharing a household with a disabled person least likely to receive support from the home help (Arber *et al.*, 1988; Parker and Lawton, 1991a).

Carers sometimes face problems arising from the limited tasks that home care workers undertake. Elderly carers can often manage light cleaning, but want help with washing paintwork, gardening, taking down curtains and other heavy duty work that is sometimes regarded as unnecessary or beyond the competence of the home help. Similarly some carers, particularly wives, want help with 'male' household tasks, such as mending fuses and putting up shelves, that their husbands can no longer do (Parker, 1992). Because the home care service is modelled on female domestic labour, it does not undertake such work and there is no easily available alternative service that does. Service planners need to give more attention to how these forms of help could be provided.

The timing of the service can also pose problems. Many home care services still only operate from nine to one, and they will rarely guarantee the exact time that a worker will call. This poses problems for carers who work and would like someone to get the person they look after up, dressed and perhaps ready for the transport to day care. Similar problems arise at the end of the day. These limitations mean that home care is of little use to most working carers.

Home care can also be unreliable. Twigg and Atkin describe the constant instability of home help allocations due to sickness, holidays and the pressure on resources. Cases where carers are involved are particularly prone to suffer from such instability since they are perceived to be less vulnerable than clients who are wholly unsupported. From the perspective of the home care organiser juggling the cases is a triumph of personnel effort and skill, but from that of the carers it means that they never know whether someone is coming that week, or whether sickness and holidays will result in temporary withdrawal, often unannounced. Again as a result, some carers feel the service is more trouble than it is worth.

The home care service can also suffer from a rather narrow approach to assessment. Home care organisers have traditionally existed in a separate world from other service providers. Their contacts with other services tend to be limited, and sometimes made unrewarding by feelings of professional inferiority (Sinclair et al., 1990; Twigg and Atkin, 1993). Organisers have often had little training or encouragement to go beyond simply assessing for their service, and they are not always well equipped to see other problems or solutions. This matters in relation to carers because the home care service is the predominant form of help that elderly people receive. Few come into contact with a social worker, so that if the carer has special needs, it is up to the home care service to recognise and act upon them. Assessment skills and better integration with other services are thus important training needs for home care organisers.

The home care service is changing. It is increasingly subject to a more managed approach, with attempts over the last decade to move it away from the traditional thin-spread model, in which the majority of allocations are for two hours a week, towards a thick-spread one, where coverage is at higher intensity but for fewer people. Home helps have at the same time had to adopt more flexible forms of working and provide personal care as well as – and increasingly instead of – housework (SSI, 1987a, 1987b, 1988). Personal care has traditionally been provided by the home help service on an idiosyncratic and often personalised basis (Twigg, 1990). It has been difficult to determine whether it is available in a locality. Moves towards a more focused service have emphasised this aspect of the work; though the extent of the shift is still unclear.

The move towards a more intensively targeted service has implications for carers. It is likely, in the context of the withdrawal of service from the lighter end of disability, that the current biases in allocation against those who share a house or have a relative nearby will continue and even intensify; unless, that is, the needs of carers are added explicitly to the priorities of the service. This has happened in certain authorities, often in association with attempts to clarify and prioritise in more complex ways which clients should receive the service. Intervention targets have been developed in which the needs of highly stressed carers have been included in an overall matrix of priorities. How common these developments will become remains to be seen.

To summarise:

- The home care service has traditionally been targeted in such a way as not to support carers. This is despite the fact that there is clear evidence of its relevance, particularly to the situation of carers who share a household with someone with dementia.

- Carers sometimes want help with tasks that home care staff do not undertake, like spring cleaning, gardening or male household tasks. Personal care is sometimes available from the home care service, but not always. It is often provided on an idiosyncratic, individual basis.

- Some carers need help at the beginning and end of the day, and thus have difficulties with the current limited hours.

- Home care allocations can be unstable and cannot always be relied upon. Carers in particular lose out in this regard.

- Home care organisers do not always make sufficiently full assessments, and this can lead to their missing the needs of carers.

- Moves towards a more concentrated service are likely to disadvantage carers further, unless their needs are explicitly incorporated into the priorities of the service.

Medical services: general practitioners

General practitioners are the only service providers with whom the majority of the population is in contact; and they are, therefore, potentially central in the recognition of the needs of carers and the mobilisation of help for them. Although GPs are held in high esteem in the population in general, studies of carers have detected a more equivocal note. Lewis and Meredith (1988) found that GPs: 'received the worst press from our carers'. Twigg and Atkin (1993) found more variable views, with some carers describing their GP as supportive and informative, but others as brusque and ill-informed.

Levin and her colleagues (1989) and Wright (1986) reported a majority of carers (between a half and two-thirds) as finding the GP helpful. In Wright's study a favourable assessment was particularly associated with a willingness to undertake home visits. Levin et al.'s supporters valued GPs for the security and confidence they gave as well as for their more directly medical expertise. There is also some evidence that younger GPs who have undergone the new professional training are more sympathetic to the needs of carers (Parker, 1992; Twigg and Atkin, 1993); and this may also apply to women GPs (Parker, 1992).

Levels of contact with carers vary. Overall, 22 per cent of carers in the OPCS survey of carers reported that the person they looked after was in regular contact with the GP (defined as at least once a month). Among those who shared a household with the cared-for person, the level was 13 per cent; and among those who did not (mostly the carers of older people) it was 26 per cent (Green, 1988). For those sharing a household, the GP was the service provider they were most commonly in contact with; for those not sharing a household, the GP came second to the home help (Green, 1988). Levin and her colleagues in their study of supporters of elderly people with confusion found that half of the carers had spoken to a GP about their relative in the last three months. No clear pattern emerged in relation to the physical disability or mental state of the patient, though there was some evidence that the GP became involved at the point of deterioration of the older person or of their domestic situation.

Twigg and Atkin argue that general practitioners' awareness of the carer's situation is often limited by the way they practise. General practitioners largely operate on the basis of demand, responding to individual consultations initiated by the patient. Their perception of the situation is framed and limited by the consulting room. Many carers remain literally invisible to the GP because they never attend the surgery or because the cared-for person goes alone into the consulting room. This is particularly characteristic of the carers of people with mental health problems or of certain forms of chronic illness or physical disability where the cared-for person is well able to manage the interchange with the doctor, and where arguably it is quite appropriate for them to do so. Some GPs only become aware of the existence of a carer when they call at the house for an emergency; it is only then that the wider social situation of the patient and the possible needs of the carer become apparent. There are obvious implications here for the use of over-75 assessment visits as a means of identifying carers and their needs.

General practitioners are under severe time constraint imposed by the pace of consultation. There is rarely time in the few minutes allowed to explore the wider situation of the patient. This is a familiar difficulty in general practice, but it has particular implications for carers, who are often reluctant to assert their needs, and fall easily into a mode of consultation in which everything focuses on the needs of the cared-for person (Twigg and Atkin, 1993). Carers have to be very assertive and self-confident to shift attention to their needs. The traditional bias in medicine towards a narrow focus on the patient – and sometimes only on the condition – reinforces this tendency. General practitioners tend to define the problem first in medical terms and secondly in terms of the individual patient (Jewson, 1976; Armstrong, 1983; Brisenden, 1987) and this leaves little room for the carer in the consultation.

General practitioners are variable in the degree to which they give information to the carer about the condition and its likely course. Some carers in Twigg and Atkin's study reported that the GP was helpful and they felt supported by his or her advice and information. Some, however, felt left in the dark; and this appeared particularly so in relation to senile dementia and schizophrenia. In Levin and her colleagues' study of dementia (1989), two-fifths of the supporters had had no explanation from the doctor as to what was wrong with their relative. This lack of information about the condition partly appears to relate to pressure of time, but it seems to arise also from an emotional reluctance of some medical practitioners to address directly the needs of people who are not going to get well. Neither dementia nor schizophrenia has an optimistic prognosis, and GPs sometimes seemed reluctant to discuss this with carers. Of course, it is not always easy to predict the exact course of an illness; and this difficulty is compounded in the case of conditions like multiple sclerosis that are fluctuating by nature. General practitioners sometimes express concern lest they provide information too soon, in advance of the situation to be coped with or in a way that might distress or depress the carer (Twigg and Atkin, 1993). Though Levin and her colleagues did report some cases where the carer was distressed by information offered by the doctor, the commoner response was one of gratitude. Carers in general value knowing more about the condition and its likely course. They find it enables them to come to terms with the situation and to adjust their expectations of the cared-for person. The latter point is particularly helpful in relation to conditions like dementia and schizophrenia where the cared-for person is not always responsible for his or her behaviour but where it can be disturbing or hurtful unless seen as part of the illness.

Difficulties can sometimes arise when the carer and the cared-for person have different GPs. This applies most commonly where they do not share a household. Even where they share a GP, there can still be problems over confidentiality. Carers can experience frustration at the refusal of the GP to discuss their relative's condition. Issues of confidentiality arise in particular in relation to mental health problems like depression where GPs can be particularly concerned to protect the privacy of the patient, and this privacy can extend to spouses (Twigg and Atkin, 1993). Issues of patient confidentiality are, however, real ones that require a sensitive balancing of the two interests.

General practitioners often lack any formal training in relation to the social dimensions of their work. As a result they tend either to avoid responding in these areas, or do so on the basis of 'common sense' assumptions deriving from their own social worlds. The variable and often idiosyncratic response of GPs has been widely commented upon. Twigg and Atkin found that GPs were in general not unsympathetic to carers, but that they sometimes applied rather stereotypical ideas about, for example, the roles of men and women, or the 'virtuous' nature of certain carers, and this meant that they sometimes accepted the nature of the situation and did not explore ways in which the carer's position might be improved.

General practitioners are often ignorant about other local services and rarely have any systematic method for finding out about them. The reluctance of doctors to refer to social services is well established (Mechanic, 1970; Ellard, 1974; Borne and Lewis, 1977; Huntingdon, 1981). Links with social service departments tend to be poor, and contact with the voluntary sector patchy. Carers, however, trust GPs to be knowledgeable, and assume that if they have not been told about some form of support or service, it does not exist.

General practitioners' expectations of being in command make it difficult for them to refer to services over which they have no direct control. This applies in particular to social services and the voluntary sector. As a result they prefer to refer to services in the health sector, ideally those directly under their control (Huntingdon, 1981; Wilkin, quoted in Sinclair et al., 1990; Twigg and Atkin, 1993). This has consequences for carers, whose needs tend to be primarily in the social rather than health sphere.

To summarise:

- General practitioners occupy a pivotal position in community care. They are the first port of call for many carers who are otherwise not linked into service support. They are, however, variable in their responses, particularly in relation to social aspects, where they have little training.

- Carers are unaware of this variability and assume that everything that is available has been reviewed and offered.

- The way GPs practise, in a consulting room and under pressure, means that carers often remain invisible to them. The focus of medicine is on the patient, and carers have to be very assertive to move that focus on to themselves.

- Carers value information about the condition of the person they look after, and GPs are particularly well placed to give this. The issue of confidentiality needs to be addressed with sensitivity, recognising the interests of both carer and cared for.

- General practitioners are often ignorant about local services, and their expectations of command can mean they prefer to refer within the health sector. Many of the most important forms of support for carers, however, are found outside the health sector. General practitioners need to be more proactive in making such inter-sectoral referrals.

Hospital based doctors

Hospital based doctors are not normally included in reviews of the workings of community care. They are not based in the community, and the specialist nature of their work means that their remit tends to be more narrowly medical than is the case with GPs. However, as Twigg and Atkin argue, hospital consultants can play a significant role in the lives of carers: some conditions are effectively managed from the hospital; decisions made in the hospital can have direct implications for the carer; and certain specialisms, such as geriatrics and psychiatry, increasingly regard themselves as having a community dimension. It is convenient for the purposes of this review to divide hospital doctors into three broad groups – consultants in physical medicine, geriatricians and psychiatrists – and to focus mainly on the role of the consultant.

A significant number of sick and disabled people with conditions like rheumatism, back problems, diabetes and respiratory diseases are cared for primarily under the direction of a consultant in physical medicine. Their general practitioner may be involved, but to a lesser degree, with the primary management being undertaken by the hospital. This is true of the younger age groups, but applies also to older people, only some of whom come under the care of a geriatrician. For the carers of these patients, the hospital consultant can play an important role.

The process of hospital discharge illustrates the way in which the decisions of consultants can have importance for carers. Hospital discharge has been identified as a time of stress and difficulty for many carers who have to deal with new responsibilities and changed relationships. Sometimes the return from hospital is accompanied by a considerable load of physical nursing that falls on the carer (Parker, 1992). Additional problems can arise when the hospital doctor making the decision about discharge fails to consult the carer, simply assuming his or her presence and ability to care. This is particularly a problem on those acute wards where there is no tradition of discharge planning and little in the way of machinery to ensure that the needs of the patient and the carer are explored. Here the actions of the consultant can have a very direct effect on the life of the carer. All too often carers are simply assumed to be able to cope.

Although consultants are potentially significant figures in the lives of carers, the way in which they practise means that they are not always aware of carers. The limitation of view imposed by the process of consultation referred to above in relation to GPs is even more acute in relation to hospital doctors who, moreover, rarely if ever visit patients in their home circumstances. As a result carers remain literally invisible to many of these doctors. Consultants in physical medicine also tend to adopt a narrower view of their remit, emphasising the medical nature of their specialism. Their focus is on the patient, and often only on his or her specific condition, and the wider situation is not seen as part of their responsibility. It is important to emphasise that this narrowness of view can be entirely appropriate. The input of the consultant is specialist, and he or she has little or no training or expertise in wider social aspects. Problems arise however where the consultant is the *only* service provider with whom the carer or the cared-for person is in contact. Then they can assume a particularly significant role, but it is one that they may be unaware of, or unwilling to act upon.

In general the traditions of geriatric medicine are broader. The needs of carers are perceived to be part of the care equation of older people. The role of carers in hospital discharge is recognised, at least in theory. The routes into contact with the geriatrician for those living in the community are, however, sometimes unclear. Levin and her colleagues failed to find any association between likelihood of contact with the geriatrician and any features or problems of the carer. Two-fifths of those who had had contact with a geriatrician found him or her helpful; but one-fifth did not. Only two-fifths of those in contact had had their relative's mental condition explained to them. As with general practitioners, carers found such information helpful even where distressing. Carers also valued geriatricians for their ability to open doors to other forms of medical support.

People diagnosed as mentally ill are largely cared for within a medical context, and consultant psychiatrists are key figures in the management of their support (Perring et al., 1990). In Twigg and Atkin's study, the psychiatrists marginalised carers less than did the consultants in physical medicine. They were more likely to have met the carer and regarded doing so as important. It was clear, however, that the significance they attached to this related less to the potential needs of the carer than to the wish to gain more information about the background of the patient. In general psychiatrists showed sympathy for carers, but their practice remained largely focused on the patient. Carers tended to feature as 'family' or 'relatives' – part of the social and emotional background of the patient – rather than as carers with needs in their own right.

To summarise:

- Carers whose only contact is with acute hospital care often find themselves linked into a service that is not attuned to their needs and which may be unaware of their existence.

- Consultant psychiatrists tend to be more aware of the existence of carers, but their practice remains strongly focused on the patient.

Community nursing service

A number of writers have argued for the potential significance of the community nursing service in the support of carers (Robinson, 1988; Nolan and Grant, 1989; Atkinson and McHaffie, 1992; Atkinson, 1992). Nurses are relevant to a range of problems faced by carers. In addition to skilled nursing input, they can give advice and help about the course and management of medical conditions; they can help with incontinence and bathing and other forms of personal care; they can listen and encourage; they can give information and refer. Since they go into the home and observe over time, they are in a better position than, for example, general practitioners to be aware of the existence of a carer and of potential strains.

In general, this potential has not been realised. Even where support for carers is recognised as an appropriate aim of the service, it is easily displaced by the pressures of crisis intervention and technical medical tasks. Although the community nursing service, particularly in the context of more holistic models of nurse training, is concerned with the well-being of the patient in the widest sense, and this includes their family circumstances, the realities are that nurses are still quite closely task-oriented, with priority being given to specific medical interventions.

Those carers who do receive the support of nurses are full of their praise, valuing in particular the practical, hands-on help they give, often with tasks that the carers find physically difficult or embarrassing (Wright, 1986; Lewis and Meredith, 1988; Levin et al., 1989). The main problem for carers appears to be one of limited access. Four areas of shortfall have been identified. First, carers undertake tasks that can be regarded as more appropriate for a nurse – such as septic dressings, injections and manual evacuation of bowels. A number of studies have described cases where nursing support would by any professional judgement have been appropriate, but where it was not provided (Levin *et al.*, 1989; Atkinson, 1992; Parker, 1992). Many carers thus struggle with nursing tasks that are onerous or embarrassing for them. Sometimes this results from a lack of knowledge of the service or of how to access it. But sometimes it results from the response of nurses; and some carers have reported pressure from nurses to undertake tasks such as injections that they felt that it was more appropriate for a trained nurse to do – a form of reverse substitution that they resent (Twigg and Atkin, 1993).

The second area of shortfall is in relation to personal care. Here the appropriateness of the involvement of nurses is less clear cut. Personal care falls on the boundary between tasks of a clearly nursing character that are commonly regarded as requiring a trained nurse and the simpler tasks of home nursing that lay people are accustomed to undertake. Personal care, however, involves nakedness, touching, contact with excreta, and as such borders on areas of taboo or social constraint (Ungerson, 1983; Twigg, 1990). Some carers – and indeed the recipients of care also – experience embarrassment and difficulty in these areas, and would welcome help from the community nursing service. Some carers are also, through their own frailty or disability, unable to help in these areas. It is far from clear, however, whether carers can expect help with these tasks from the community nursing service. Community nurses, particularly auxiliaries, do give what are often termed 'social baths', and they will sometimes help get a patient up and dressed, but the basis for their doing so is undefined and shifts according to pressure on individual case loads (Twigg, 1990). As a result it is difficult for carers to get a definitive answer as to whether such help is available. Certainly many carers who would like help do not receive it; and Levin and her colleagues found that two–fifths of those caring for someone with dementia who experienced difficulty giving personal care had not been offered help. There are also reasons to think that pressure on resources over the last decade has led to a withdrawal of the service from these areas.

Incontinence is widely recognised to be a particularly difficult problem for carers to manage; and its presence has been implicated in the breakdown of informal care (Gilhooly, 1986; Blannin, 1987; Hagan, 1989). A number of studies have identified the shortfall in advice and support in this area. Even where carers are in contact with the community nursing service, the problem does not always receive adequate attention. This is despite the fact that there is evidence that contact with the community nursing service can mitigate the stress imposed by incontinence (Levin *et al.*, 1989). Pressure on budgets also means that carers sometimes suffer from supplies being restricted on an arbitrary basis (Twigg and Atkin, 1993).

Lastly there are certain skills, such as lifting, where carers would benefit greatly from advice and training. Studies have identified the difficulties and damage that carers experience in these areas (Nolan and Grant, 1989). Few, however, receive advice. This is partly because nurses are not always alert to the need to educate carers; but also because there are significant numbers of carers who are not in contact with the community nursing service at all. This brings us on the question of which carers get help and why.

Twigg and Atkin (1993) have explored some of the bases on which nursing help is given to carers, and they identify the significance of what they term the 'focal intervention'. Nurses recognise a range of ways in which they can help carers, and, by and large see this as a legitimate part of their work; but these forms of help are usually only activated where there is a focal intervention of an acute medical type, for example an injection to be given or a dressing to be changed. Without such a focal intervention, the nurse does not call and the wider more holistic approach is not brought into play. Help with personal care in the form of bathing does not normally constitute such an intervention, and with growing pressure on resources, leading to cut backs in these areas, is unlikely to do so in the future.

Although carers in general view nurses with favour, some problems have been identified. Nurses are not always reliable in coming. Carers needs tend to be afforded low priority, and are often displaced on a crowded shift by technical interventions. Carers do not always know whether the nurse will come that day, or indeed any day. As a result some carers view the service as more trouble than it is worth (Lewis and Meredith, 1988; Badger et al., 1989, Twigg and Atkin, 1993).

Lastly, certain changes within the district nursing service have implications for carers. There is a growing tendency, under pressure of resources as well as clarification of objectives, for the district nursing service to withdraw from the area of 'social baths'. A large – though unquantified – proportion of these baths go to people who are 'unsupported'; some, however, go to assist carers, many of whom value the service. Withdrawal from this activity is likely to make their circumstances harder. Changes are also occurring in relation to skill mix. The employment of auxiliaries as well as trained nurses has long been a feature of the service (Dunnell and Dobbs, 1982); but nurses are increasingly working in more finely graded teams where assessment and hands-on care are to some degree separated (Lightfoot, 1992). The significance for carers of this trend is unclear.

The section above has largely been concerned with the work of district nurses. The community nursing service, however, also encompasses health visitors. Evidence of the involvement of health visitors with carers is slight. The remit of the health visitor has always been wider than that of the district nurse, and has tradition-ally included a more social dimension (Robinson, 1985; Dingwall, *et al.*, 1988). As a result, work with carers potentially falls within their scope. In practice, however, the health visiting service is still largely concerned with mothers and babies and with the under-fives. Though there has for many years been talk of a greater role in rela-tion to older people, this has not, by and large, been realised (Goodwin, 1988). The persistent focus on child care means that health visitors are rarely in contact with carers, except of course where the 'carers' are parents of young children.

Lastly, although practice nurses are not technically part of the community nursing service, the growth in their numbers, which have doubled in the last five years (DH, 1991), and their involve-ment in over-75 assessments mean that they have an important potential role to play in the identification of carers' needs. Whether they in fact play such a role is unknown.

To summarise:

- The community nursing service is recognised as having a role to play in the support of carers. Nurses are valued by carers and can relieve them of tasks that many find difficult.

- The main difficulty is one of shortfall in provision in relation to skilled nursing tasks, personal care, support with incontinence and training in techniques like lifting. Carers sometimes find the nursing service unreliable.

- The emphasis by health visitors on the under-fives means that they are rarely involved with carers. Practice nurses are poten-tially significant in identifying the needs of some carers.

Day respite

Day care is provided in a range of venues and forms. At one end of the spectrum, it merges into the world of lunch clubs, over-50 groups and drop-in centres; at the other, in the form of the day hos-pital, it represents an outreach of hospital services. In this section, we will cover only those facilities that have an institutional base, and where places are in some sense allocated; and our concern with day care is limited to its role in the support of carers, though we will note in passing its significance in the support of the cared-for person also. We shall at this point exclude flexible forms of day relief provided in the home to support carers. These will be covered in the next chapter.

Most day care is provided either in the social-services or voluntary sector, sometimes in purpose-built centres but also in temporary venues like church halls. Provision is mainly for older people, though some areas have specialist centres for younger physically disabled people. Day care for people with dementia is sometimes provided in specialist centres; although many day centres for older people accept attenders who have some degree of confusion. Day care for people with learning disabilities is provided in adult training centres (ATCs), sometimes renamed day centres, and in educational placements (Carter, 1981; Evans *et al.*, 1986; Seed, 1988; Tester, 1989; Sinclair *et al.*, 1990; Brearley and Mandelstram, 1992). Day centres or day hospitals are also provided for younger people with mental health problems, but these rarely if ever see themselves as providing respite for carers.

Sometimes day care is provided in residential homes, both public and private. Such day care is often of poor quality, with the older person doing no more than joining others in the lounge. It is often an alienating experience, and can cause friction with permanent residents (Fennell *et al.*, 1981; Allen, 1983). From the carer's point of view the chief advantage of such provision is that it can provide greater flexibility, particularly in relation to evenings and the beginning and end of the day when designated day centres are closed (Weaver *et al.*, 1985).

Day hospitals tend to put less emphasis – at least officially – on the support of relatives than do centres run by social services departments or the voluntary sector. Day hospitals were originally developed as a more efficient and effective setting for treatment and rehabilitation than that provided on in-patient wards (Brocklehurst and Tucker, 1980; Fennell *et al.*, 1981). Their curative and rehabilitative focus is often subverted, however, by the long-term, essentially social needs of many patients. Among these are the needs of carers. Where there is no adequate alternative socially-oriented provision, day hospitals find it difficult to escape from some element of this role.

Providing such long-term, socially-based support is more accepted in the psychogeriatric sector, and here the support of relatives is recognised as a major function (Gilleard *et al.*, 1984; Smith and Cantley, 1985). Day hospitals often accept clients whose level of dementia or behavioural problems mean they cannot be coped with at other centres. It is not always the case, however, that attendance patterns reflect such a continuum of care; and they can also arise out of particular pathways into the different service sectors, with health care staff referring within their own sector.

There is ample evidence that carers value day care both for the relief it can bring and for the opportunities it gives for them to get out or pursue tasks at home (Keegan, 1984; Smith and Cantley, 1985; Wright, 1986; Twigg and Atkin, 1993). It is particularly highly praised by the carers of people with dementia; and there is some evidence that it may enhance the objectively measured well-being of these carers (Gilleard et al., 1984; Levin et al., 1989). What is less clear is that it prevents the institutional admission of the cared-for person. Day care appears at best to delay this eventuality. Fennell and his colleagues, among others, have questioned the use of day care for clients who are on the margins of admission, arguing that the relief it gives needs to be set against the costs to carers of maintaining a situation that is essentially at crisis point.

The availability of day care varies greatly between localities, and carers are often confused about what is provided locally and by whom. Lack of co-ordination between health, social services and voluntary agencies often results in uneven provision. Rural areas pose particular problems, though attempts have been made to meet these difficulties through the use of travelling day centres (Evans et al., 1986; Tester, 1989).

Beyond this, it is clear that the amount of day relief that carers receive is closely dependent on the client-group status of the person they look after, with high levels – usually five days a week – being provided for people with learning disabilities through the ATCs and low levels – typically one day a week – for people with physical disabilities. Carers of severely mentally infirm people sometimes get as much as five days a week respite, but lower levels are more common. In the case of learning disability, the focus of the service is strongly on the client and on an educational model of provision. This emphasis is reversed in relation to dementia where day care is recognised as being primarily for the relief of the carer. Between these poles of – potentially – high provision, the focus is more mixed with an expectation that day care will benefit the disabled person as well as the carer. As we have noted, levels of provision here are typically low, and the service a very thinly spread one (Twigg and Atkin, 1993). Many carers would like more day care, and this is particularly the case with those carers of people with dementia who are receiving only one or two days a week (Levin et al., 1989; Twigg and Atkin, 1993).

Sometimes problems arise less from the level of allocation than from the unwillingness of the cared-for person to go to the centre. This can be a particular problem with younger disabled people where provision is often unattractive, lacking real stimulation and provided in a paternalistic way that reinforces a culture of dependence (Parker, 1992; Brearley and Mandelstram, 1992). It is not surprising that many disabled adults do not want to attend such places, and carers, particularly spouses, are often loath to insist on their needs in the face of such feelings. Day care, particularly for anyone who is not severely mentally impaired, must be made attractive to the attender, if it is to be successful in supporting the carer.

The boundaries of the centre often circumscribe the view of service personnel. Managers and staff rarely go outside the centre, and they often rely on an initial assessment visit by a social worker for their knowledge of the existence or otherwise of a carer. Even where they see support for carers as part of their aims, centres rarely make any systematic attempt to be in contact, relying on carers to take the initiative (Carter, 1981; Smith and Cantley, 1986). Sometimes staff with activities to organise do not see talking to carers as a priority, and sometimes they are discouraged from doing so (Fennell *et al.*, 1981). Many carers would like to have more contact with staff, with a chance to discuss how their relative is, as well as a sympathetic ear for their own difficulties. Centre staff who do provide this, sometimes on the telephone, are much valued.

Although centres are often criticised for being cut off from other services, where they do operate as a focal point for a particular client group they can be very successful in linking carers into services. Day hospitals for people with dementia, for example, can provide an important contact point and one that continues over time. If operated in a proactive way, with outreach staff, they can pick up difficulties or changes in the circumstances of carers. Adult training centres can similarly act as the focal point of learning disability services. The fact that they offer contact over time can be particularly significant in negotiating the acceptance of respite. Many carers are reluctant to accept respite, and need to be persuaded over time that it is appropriate and legitimate. Centres that are in contact over time, particularly for younger people with physical or learning disabilities, can be successful in achieving this (Twigg and Atkin, 1993).

One of the limitations in the usefulness of day care for carers is the length of the day. Usually only open from 10.30 am to 3.30 pm, they offer what Murphy (1985) rather scornfully terms 'mid-day care'. This short day is acceptable to many carers, particularly those who are themselves elderly and who only want a relatively brief break to accomplish a limited set of things. But for anyone who wants to go out for the day, attend an afternoon event, or – most significantly – undertake paid work, such provision is useless. The lack of evening or weekend provision can also be limiting for carers who want to develop a social life. Some centres are open for longer hours, particularly those that are community facilities with a recreational focus that continues in the evening. This extended day can give the carer important flexibility, and may allow him or her to take a job. Some specialist centres for people with dementia also operate on a seven day a week basis, and this can be much valued by carers.

Carers often find closures difficult to bear, a fact that again testifies to the value of the service. Long periods of closure when statutory days are added to Bank Holidays pose a particular strain.

Sometimes staff fail to inform carers directly of closures, and this can cause anger and disappointment (Twigg and Atkin, 1993).

Perhaps the most frustrating aspect of day care for carers is the unreliability of transport. Often it fails to collect clients on time, and returns them at any time between 2.30 and 4.30 pm. The unpredictability of the service eats seriously into the carer's day and causes considerable frustration. As a result, some carers opt out of the service, and many prefer to take their relative themselves (Lewis and Meredith, 1988). Collection routes can also be long, and may involve the client sitting on the bus for up to an hour. Access to day care can sometimes become a question of assessment for transport rather than assessment for the service; and those carers who are willing to bring their relative can find that a place will be made available. The problems of transport have been identified repeatedly in studies of day care (Sinclair et al., 1991). It is unclear whether they are in fact solvable. There are some indications that where the problem is given priority, as is more often the case with young disabled adults or people with learning disability, a better service can be provided. This may however be at considerable cost; and transport already represents up to a third of the cost of day care (Fennell et al., 1981).

There is some evidence that certain clients are considered 'too bad for day care' and are returned to the sole care of their families (Lewis and Meredith, 1988). Some centres cannot cope with regular incontinence or violent behaviour. There are also practice issues as to the appropriateness of mixing clients with these problems with those who are mentally alert and whose behaviour is not disturbed (Fennell et al., 1981; Brearley and Mandelstram, 1992). Whatever the merits of the various views on this, it is clear that each area should at least aim to have a range of provision so that no carer is left with the sole charge of someone who is deemed to be beyond the tolerance of an employed worker.

Finally there are particular issues concerning day care raised by new developments in the field of learning disability. Services for people with learning disability have undergone a sea change in philosophy; and this has had consequences for their carers. Progressive models of support, as are described in Chapter Two, seek to enhance the independence of the client, pursuing a goal of normalisation that emphasises integration into the community rather than segregation. In relation to ATCs and day centres, this means moving away from an unstimulating regime of contract work and low level entertainment towards more focused, high quality input, often involving activity in the community, and work on a one-to-one or small group basis. The importance of the physical setting is downgraded; and in some approaches it is regarded as having no role to play.

This new pattern of provision has major implications for carers (Brearley and Mandelstram, 1992; Twigg and Atkin, 1993). High quality, focused input means fewer hours of activity. As a result, carers can no longer rely on five days a week respite, and this can have serious consequences, particularly when the carers are having to live with challenging behaviour. Anxieties over safety can also be raised once the security provided by the centre has been lost and provision fragmented in the community. Day services for people with learning disability need to strike a fine balance between the legitimate fears of parents and the wish to allow clients to develop independence. 'Progressive' services need to acknowledge that they have a role in supporting carers, and this may appropriately mean providing them with some day respite.

To summarise:

- Day care is valued by carers, and may help enhance their mental well-being. It is particularly valuable where the cared-for person has dementia or exhibits behavioural problems.

- Availability varies greatly between localities and client groups.

- Carers sometimes find it difficult to persuade the cared-for person to attend a centre. Making provision attractive to the attender is a vital element in providing effective support for the carer.

- Despite their acknowledged role in supporting carers, centres rarely make any systematic attempt to make contact. Such contacts as occur are valued. Centres can play an important role as a continuing point of contact for services. This is particularly the case with psychogeriatric services or services for people with learning disabilities.

- Short hours, closures and transport difficulties all pose problems for carers and limit the benefits of day care.

- 'Progressive' models of day care that fragment provision can pose problems for some carers.

Overnight respite in institutions

A variety of terms are used to describe respite in institutions: rotational care, intermittent care, phased care, short-term or relief care. The main distinction turns on the degree to which the provision is frequent and cyclical or intermittent and *ad hoc*. The majority of provision is the latter, with most carers receiving spells of one or two weeks a year (Allen, 1983; Levin *et al.*, 1989). Flexible forms of respite provided on a non-institutional basis are described in Chapter Four.

Respite is available in relation to a range of client groups. The principal exception is people with mental health problems. Here the concept is notably lacking, though carers of people diagnosed as schizophrenic have expressed a wish for such a service (Twigg and Atkin, 1993). Respite is most commonly used by carers of older people, particularly those with dementia, or of children and adults with congenital physical or learning disabilities. With older people its purpose is almost entirely to give relief to carers; with younger clients it often has a more developmental focus, with the long-term aim of encouraging greater independence.

Respite is provided in a number of institutional settings: local authority homes and hostels; private residential homes and voluntary sector facilities; acute and long-stay hospitals. Respite places are not always designated as such. Respite can sometimes be 'created' out of marginal resources when a bed in a home or ward becomes temporarily vacant and is allocated on that basis. Hospital consultants and GPs with direct access to beds sometimes use them in this way on a discretionary and unrecorded basis (Packwood, 1980; Twigg and Atkin, 1993). As a result it is not always possible to say whether and how much respite is available in a locality, or what the criteria for its use are. This can pose problems for carers in gaining access to the service.

Evidence of the value of respite is clear. Carers praise it, and see it as significant in their ability to cope (Allen, 1983; Levin *et al.*, 1989; Boldy and Kuh, 1984; Levin and Moriarty, 1990; Twigg and Atkin, 1993). There is some evidence that, in conjunction with day care, with which it is strongly associated, it can reduce the carers' levels of stress (Levin *et al.*, 1989). Evidence that it can prevent institutionalisation is more equivocal. Levin and her colleagues found that the use of respite was *positively* associated with admission, but this may have been as a result of its use as a stop-gap by individuals who had expressed a wish for the older person to be admitted. Other work, however, has highlighted the fears of some carers that if they once experience the relaxation of respite they will be unable to take up the burden again (Lewis and Meredith, 1988; Scharlach and Frenzel, 1986). Donaldson and his colleagues' study (1988), however, suggests that respite *can* prevent admission where provided in a specialised context that emphasises that aim.

Respite, for all its benefits, can be a problematic service for carers. It is widely recognised as central to their support, and yet is regarded by them with some ambivalence. What are the sources of this? Respite presents more sharply than any other service the potential conflict of interest between the carer and the cared-for person. The idea of going into an institution, however temporarily, is disliked by many disabled people, and carers understandably do not want to force the issue. As a result respite is relatively rarely taken up where the cared-for person is mentally alert, or where he or she is cared for by a spouse. Only six per cent of the elderly people in Allen's study of respite in residential homes were cared for by spouses (Allen, 1983). Parker (1992) has explored the tensions that arise in marriages when respite is proposed. Whose interests predominate draws on the dynamics of power in the relationship; and sometimes these reflect structural expectations in relation to gender, with women less likely to press their interests than men. Lewis and Meredith in their study of mothers and daughters also found that the long-established dynamics of relationships were significant in determining whose interests had priority (Lewis and Meredith, 1988).

In general, the more that the experience can be made a positive one for the cared-for person, the easier it is to get the carer to accept respite. Where the cared-for person is a young person living at home, respite, if well handled, can be a means of encouraging independence and widening social horizons. Among older people, particularly those with dementia, it is harder to find a genuinely rehabilitative aspect, and the chief concern must be to make the period away as little damaging as possible.

Barriers to uptake can arise from fear of the deterioration of the cared-for person in respite. Such anxieties are in part borne out by research. Elderly people can become more confused, and their behaviour and health decline as a result of respite (Kelson, 1985; Rai *et al.*, 1986; Wright, 1986). Carers sometimes say that the effort of getting the person back to their previous state means that the break is not worth having (Wright, 1986). Levin and her colleagues argue, however, that respite can be reformed in such a way as to minimise these effects.

Carers sometimes find it hard to accept respite because they have no one with whom to share the break that it gives them. Caring can be an isolating experience, and many carers find that they no longer have anyone with whom they can enjoy themselves or go on holiday. The problem is particularly acute for spouse carers. Many carers make their lives so much around caring that they cannot conceive of a break, or have not the energy to accept one. Some carers refuse respite until they reach breaking point when it is forced on them by circumstances. In these cases, however, they often come to value the service and wish they had accepted it earlier (Twigg and Atkin, 1993).

What such barriers point to is the importance of the sensitive negotiation of the service. It is not enough simply to suggest respite to carers. They need to be encouraged to use it, to have their anxieties allayed and permission given. This can take time. Those services or service providers that remain in contact with the carer over time are in a better position to achieve this; and for this reason services that provide a focal point, such as the day centre or hospital, are particularly successful routes into respite.

There are a number of other ways in which respite could be made more attractive and acceptable to carers. Quality issues need to be addressed. The poor level of much provision, in run-down facilities with inadequate staffing, can be a serious barrier to acceptance. Seeing people with dementia en masse can be a depressing experience, and carers need to be helped to distinguish their feelings about this from judgements about the standard of care. However, serious issues about quality do exist, and carers can be shocked by the material, and sometimes the care, standards that pertain in some long-stay facilities. For these reasons it is particularly important that a full account be given to the carer of any incidents such as falls or bruising. Failure to do this feeds anxieties, and can lead to a carer's deciding not to use respite again. This applies to carers of people with learning disabilities as much as older people (Levin et al., 1989; Twigg and Atkin, 1993).

Some of the problems of respite relate to venue. It is clear that acute wards do not, in general, provide a good setting for respite: they are too busy; they prioritise acute medical care; and the regimes allow little attention to be given to the social needs of short–stay patients (Hasselkus and Brown, 1983; Frank, 1984). The difficulty of integrating respite care into institutions whose main purposes are different is not confined to hospitals. Large residential care homes share many of the same problems (Boldy and Kuh, 1984), and Allen reported that the heads of these homes felt that such respite was an alienating experience for most older people, and one that was disturbing to residents also. Where the older person is mentally alert there is the added distress of sharing the home with people who have dementia, and who represent a sizeable proportion of residents in homes. Distressing experiences with other residents are often reported to be the most upsetting aspect of respite (Allen, 1983).

In general, it appears that respite is best provided either in a specialist facility or as a specialist function within a larger unit where the particular needs of short-term residents and their carers can be made the main subject of concern. A number of studies have pointed to the ways in which the experience of respite can be made better for both parties: procedures to prepare the elderly or disabled person can be improved; information about them can be transmitted to make their stay less disturbing and an individual care plan prepared; contact can be maintained with the carers and their anxieties addressed; a flexible policy over visiting can be developed; and rehabilitation where appropriate attempted (Oswin, 1984; Robinson, 1987, 1988; Allen, 1983; Levin and Moriarty, 1990).

Carers sometimes face problems in gaining access to respite. Respite is strongly associated, among both older people and those with learning disabilities, with attendance at day care (Allen, 1983; Levin and Moriarty, 1990). This is not simply a product of a common underlying need for relief, but points up the importance of being networked into a service in order to receive further help (Allen, 1983). We have already noted the importance in respite of negotiating the service over time. Twigg and Atkin also found that some carers whose relative no longer attended day care but who went to some other, usually educational, placement did not receive respite though they wanted to. Where respite was provided on a one-off, marginal basis, as is often the case in hospitals where consultants allocate it at their discretion, it was particularly difficult for carers to find out about, and they found the pathways of access puzzling.

Lastly problems also arise for carers from the inflexible nature of much provision. Respite is commonly provided in units of a week, often with the change-round day on Saturday. Managers concerned to maximise occupancy are loath to break up the pattern by providing single days, or, worse, weekends that disrupt two weeks of allocation; but these are often what carers want. Carers also want the chance of emergency or last minute access for times when things get on top of them or in order to accept social opportunities as they arise. Again this sort of valued access is in conflict with maintaining high levels of occupancy.

Some at least of the difficulties recounted above can be met through more flexible forms of provision that are not confined to an institutional base. Family-based respite has become increasingly common in the field of learning disability, where it is now the preferred form. These models have increasingly been extended to older people. Both are covered in the next chapter.

To summarise:

- Institutional respite is valued by those carers that use it, and there is evidence to suggest that it improves their levels of well-being. Evidence that it prevents institutionalisation is lacking. This may however be a result of the way in which it is used.

- Respite is a service that needs careful and sensitive negotiation. Many carers feel ambivalent about accepting it. They value the break but feel guilty about using it. It is often disliked by the cared-for person, and take-up is particularly low where the cared-for person is a spouse or mentally alert.

- Other barriers to take up include: fears of deterioration; anxieties about the quality of care; and the decay of the carer's social life so that a break offers little chance of enjoyment.

- Respite appears to be most successful where provided in a specialist facility or as a specialist function in a larger unit.

- Attempts to maximise bed occupancy can lead to respite being provided in inflexible and standardised packages that do not meet the needs of individual carers.

Carer support groups

Carer support groups are one of the few forms of support that are directly provided for carers. Groups can be organised in a number of ways. Some are offshoots of a facility like a day hospital or adult training centre; others are free standing. Some are generic, open to all carers; others focus on a particular client group, even a particular medical condition. Some are very much for the carers; others have a shared emphasis on the carer and the cared-for person. Some are linked into national charities; others are strictly local. All share certain common features around the provision of mutual support and the sharing of information. The critical distinction is between groups that are organised, and to some degree controlled by professionals, and those that are genuinely in the hands of their members. In this section we shall discuss the role of groups in supporting carers. Their role in advocacy and pressure-group politics will be referred to in the final chapter.

In general research suggests that groups are valued by those who attend them (Glosser and Wexler, 1985; Hinrichsen et al., 1985). Evidence that they produce direct improvements in the well-being of carers, or in their ability to continue is however more equivocal (Toseland et al., 1992). Above all what groups offer is mutual support, the opportunity to meet people in a similar situation and to share problems and experiences in an empathetic way. Although groups can offer the opportunity for individuals to ventilate powerfully negative feelings, in general they appear to operate at a lower emotional key.

Carer support groups are also important information exchanges. Sometimes this happens in a formal way when a speaker attends to talk about some aspect of caring or of service support, but often it happens informally between members of the group. This sort of exchange can be particularly helpful since many carers are not only uncertain about what is available but also what it is appropriate to ask for help with. Hearing of the success of people in a similar situation can be encouraging. Carer groups can also be useful in enabling individuals to perceive themselves as carers; and such self-identity can help them be more assertive in seeking and accepting service support (Twigg and Atkin, 1993).

Some groups are involved in providing significant social and recreational facilities for carers. Twigg and Atkin found that the most successful groups were those that operated on this basis, often in the evenings from community centres and involving a large and sociable group of people. In all cases these were either parent groups or were attached to a recreational style day centre for physically disabled people that also operated in the evenings as a community facility. Groups run by social workers or psychiatric nurses, usually for the carers of older people, were less sociable.

Where professionals are involved or where the group is associated with a facility like a day hospital or day centre, it can act as a bridge between carers and key service providers. Carers can find such informal but regular contacts useful in discussing problems or letting practitioners know of changes in their circumstances. It is important when emphasising the benefits of such groups not to miss the advantages they bring to professionals. Smith and Cantley's account (1985) of a group attached to a psychogeriatric day hospital makes plain the ways in which the meetings were used by staff to channel and defuse individual discontent; to relieve the medical staff from demands for individual consultations; and to present an optimistic account of the cared-for person's condition and of the hospital as an active therapeutic institution.

Sometimes carers and service providers differ about the functions and benefits of the group (Twigg and Atkin, 1993). Professionals often appear to have an image of the group that derives from a therapy model, in which there is an expectation that strong feelings will be ventilated and that the group will 'work' on its problems. This can be in contrast to carers who are largely untouched by psychotherapeutic culture and who simply look to the group to provide some company. Where professionals control access to the group they are able in some degree to impose this model, suggesting that it is 'time' for certain individuals to move on or that social events should take place somewhere else. Differences can also emerge over the issue of cliques. Professionals tend to want to break these down and assert the ways in which the group is open to all; whereas attenders can see these as natural patterns of sociability. Professionals, having started a group, often want to wean it away into a self-governing mode. This can pose problems, with the attenders being unwilling to take up the responsibility either because they have been disempowered by the way the group was set up, or because that was the form that they preferred. It is much easier for a group to thrive as a self-help association if it starts on that basis.

Groups sometimes experience difficulties over recruitment. Where they are attached to a facility, this is less of a problem; but where they are free standing, whether self-help or facilitated by a professional, there is no natural feeder mechanism. Advertisements and leaflets tend to have limited impact, and this is particularly true of unfocused, blanket advertising. Carers are not easy to contact, and tend to be socially isolated. Many are unsure as to whether a group is for them. In these cases, personal invitation and encouragement can be vital. In general, self-help groups are better at providing mutual support in attending, though social workers will also sometimes accompany a new member. Wilson's book on self care groups (1986) provides useful suggestions about setting up and running a carers' group.

Some carers face practical difficulties in attending. Unless the group meets at a day centre, substitute care can be a problem, and one that may require additional resources in the form of money or volunteers. Not all carers, however, want to use their limited access to either in this way. Transport can pose problems, particularly since many carers are not young and are on low incomes. Organising shared transport can be helpful. There can also be problems of a practical kind associated with the venue. Carer support groups often have to rely on marginal resources, meeting in large, unsuitable rooms, with no facilities for refreshments. Getting a welcoming, comfortable and above all sociable venue is important for the success of a group.

Finally, carer support groups do not appeal to everyone; and it is important to recognise this. Some carers are not interested in hearing about other people's problems and struggles, feeling they have enough of their own. Others want to use the few opportunities that they have to get out to enjoy themselves and forget about caring. Some carers welcome the chance to be linked into a group through a newsletter, but do not want to attend on a regular basis. Needs can also change over time. Some carers value the chance initially to talk and unburden, but having been through that experience move on to wanting another format, emphasising perhaps the recreational or advocacy sides.

To summarise:

- Carers value support groups as an opportunity to share experiences with people in a similar situation and to exchange information and emotional support. Groups that offer a recreational aspect can be popular. Not all carers, however, want to attend a group.

- Support groups can offer an opportunity for linking the carer to facilities like day hospitals or centres.

- Carers and professionals sometimes differ over the function and benefits of the group. Carers rarely endorse the more directly therapeutic model that some professionals espouse.

The integration of services

So far we have treated the different services as discrete entities. As important as any single service, however, is they way in which they interact. Users and carers often have a variety of needs for which no single service is alone appropriate; furthermore the effectiveness of one service can depend on the provision of another. How the services are put together is central in meeting the needs of users and carers.

Evidence for the creation of complex packages of care is however lacking. The dominant account of service provision is one of fragmentation, and of the lack of comprehensive assessment and care planning that would allow for the mobilisation of an interconnected set of services. The barriers to such mobilisation are threefold: organisational, cultural and financial. Service providers have traditionally been faced with a limited range of services on which to draw; and many of these have been organised in over-bureaucratic ways that mean they are unable to respond flexibly. Inter-professional relations have been marked by distrust rooted in conflicts between medical and social accounts of the situation, but fuelled also by status differences. These cultural conflicts are not confined to the medical/social divide, but extend within their respective hierarchies also. As a result practitioners often find it difficult to work together, or to recognise each other's expertise. Separate budgets underline these divisions, and mean that assessments cannot be shared, but have to be particular to the individual service. Separate budgets also lead to attempts to off-load costs, and to other forms of 'perverse incentives' (Audit Commission, 1986; Griffiths, 1988; Hunter et al., 1988; Sinclair et al., 1990; Allen et al., 1992).

It is in the context of these problems of fragmentation that case management, or care management as it is termed in the government documentation, has increasingly been proposed. Case management was developed in the USA as a means of overcoming the fragmentation and dislocation inherent in a system that was project based, relied on multiple funding and lacked a coherent organisational focus. The case management model was brought to Britain in experimental form in the 1980s, and was particularly associated with the work of the Personal Social Services Research Unit at the University of Kent and with the Kent community care experiment. The evaluation of this and associated developments suggested that case management for elderly people on the brink of admission to a residential home could deliver a more efficient and effective response than standard services (Davies and Challis, 1986; Challis and Davies, 1986). The approach has been taken up and developed more widely in other experimental schemes (Dant and Gearing, 1990; Richardson and Higgins, 1992; Meethan and Thompson, 1992).

Under the title 'care management' this approach forms the central plank in the new community care as outlined in the 1990 NHS and Community Care Act and the associated policy and practice guidance (DH, 1990; SSI, 1991a, b, c, d). The principal advantages of

92

the approach are described in terms of: the ability to move services towards a needs-led as opposed to service-dominated approach; the provision of care planning at an individual level, specifying desirable outcomes; and the provision of a more integrated service response and one that draws on a wider range of services across the statutory, voluntary and private sectors. Throughout the government documentation, the terms 'users and carers' are consistently linked; and balancing the two sets of needs is recognised as one of the tasks of the care manager.

As yet there is no evaluative evidence as to the effectiveness of the new structures; and implementation has itself been delayed. What indications are there from earlier work on case management as to their likely impact on carers? First, there is evidence for the capacity of case management to increase the well-being of carers, though this has been subject to dispute (Davies and Challis, 1986; Parker, 1990b; Challis and Davies, 1991). Secondly, there may be a tendency in case management systems with devolved budgets to regard carers as a form of 'free good', a resource within the community whose input they can assume and therefore need not support. This is not, however, a necessary part of the approach. The needs and interests of carers can be incorporated if this is seen as appropriate and made an explicit aim of the service. Thirdly, it is clear that the professional background and institutional location of the service providers affect how far they are aware of and responsive to carers. Twigg and Atkin found that social workers and those trained in a social care model were more aware of the needs of carers than were those whose training was medical in nature; they were thus more likely to consider them as part of their assessment, though this did not necessarily lead to greater provision of help. Such differences between professionals are likely to affect care managers also.

To summarise:

- Inflexible service and a lack of integration have been identified as central problems in the provision of community care. Carers suffer from these as much as users.

- Care management offers a potential way forward, and one that can be made sensitive to the needs of carers. In order to do this agencies need to include responsiveness to carers among the explicit aims of intervention. These aims should be recorded and open for carers to read.

4

Innovations and special schemes

DIANA LEAT

What is innovation?

This chapter is concerned with innovations and with special schemes for the support of carers. The first difficulty in writing about innovations is that it is not altogether clear what counts as such. In some cases innovation is a label attached to a piece of work in order to increase its political attractiveness or its chances of securing acceptance and funding. Some of the 'innovations' described below are ten or twenty years old but are still regarded as innovative in the sense that they are not widespread, established or entirely secure in their funding. This fact alone says something important about the time it takes to become 'established' and widely accepted, and about the precarious existence of many areas of work whose value is not in dispute.

Services described as innovative do not necessarily entail anything very new. The label 'innovation' may be applied to a new way of working, or form of provision, or to an old way of doing things which happens to be new to a particular locality. Innovation may involve an old way of working with a new group or in relation to a new or previously unrecognised need; in this sense, all projects which focus specifically on the needs and perspectives of carers are innovative. Innovation may also be applied to a re-mix of old ways of working or existing provisions to create a different whole. Or, as we noted at the start of Chapter Three, it may involve a relatively minor, but from the viewpoint of users highly significant adaptation of well-established mainstream provision, such as providing day care on Saturdays or Sundays.

Identifying the range of types of innovation is important because different types involve different levels of change and risk and have different resource and management implications. Recognising that innovation does not necessarily require radical departures highlights the potential for creating something new and different from old materials or within existing resources.

Before looking at some examples of innovation in supporting carers, it is important to make some general points. First, innovation is not good *per se* but must be judged in terms of its relevance, accessibility, acceptability and reliability from the viewpoint of carers. But, as Chapter Two has demonstrated, different groups of carers have different needs, preferences, levels of tolerance and criteria for assessing acceptability. A type of provision organised in one way, in one place, at one time may be acceptable, relevant and accessible to one group but not to another. Planners and policy makers should not simply choose the type of innovation they prefer but must foster those which 'fit' the group for whom they are intended.

Secondly, it is important to put any innovation into its wider context: what may be useful, relevant, acceptable and accessible as one part of an integrated package of provision may be none of these things if provided on its own. We have touched on some of the problems of providing a comprehensive and integrated service in Chapter Three; and special schemes add another element to this. Thirdly, innovations in support of carers must be assessed in terms of carers' needs and preferences, and not solely in terms of wider policy goals or benefits to the cared-for person. As we have noted, many forms of support are primarily focused on the cared-for person. In some cases the distinction between the benefit of carers and those they care for is difficult to draw in practice; in other cases the distinction is crucial and makes a fundamental difference to the way in which the service is planned and allocated.

Fourthly, despite the widely accepted view that the role of the voluntary sector is to pioneer and innovate, the available research evidence suggests that voluntary organisations are not the only or indeed the most significant source of innovations. A study of organisations for the physically and mentally handicapped found that much of what was regarded as innovative by voluntary agencies were in fact small-scale, non-controversial, incremental improvements or extensions to existing programmes. Kramer suggested that because innovation is highly valued, especially by funders, voluntary organisations tend to emphasise innovation at the expense of other important aspects such as access and choice for users and effectiveness in performance (Kramer, 1981). One needs to be wary of the notion that 'innovation = voluntary sector' and 'voluntary sector = innovation' and to understand the distinction between substance and presentation for funding purposes.

It is also worth remembering that large voluntary organisations may find innovation difficult because of their bureaucratic mode of organisation and decision-making processes; and small ones may find it difficult because they do not have the organisational and management infrastructure to make things happen and carry them, through. The key to innovation may be the existence of 'welfare entrepreneurs' with the power and freedom to seize opportunities as they arise; a willingness to take risks is also important (Knapp, 1991; Jowell, 1991).

To summarise:

- Innovation does not necessarily entail anything very new.

- Innovation is not good *per se* but must be judged in terms of its relevance, accessibility, acceptability and reliability from the viewpoint of the carer.

- Voluntary organisations are not the only or indeed the most significant source of innovations.

Examples of innovation

Although a review of this length cannot be comprehensive, it can provide some examples of new approaches to providing support for carers, paying particular attention to initiatives which have been subjected to relatively systematic analysis and evaluation. This chapter discusses special schemes in support for carers under five main headings:

- Neighbourhood care, community care and sitting schemes

- Flexible care attendance

- Flexible respite

- Information, advice and support

- Consultation and involvement in planning

These five headings are not mutually exclusive and some specific schemes straddle the border lines; the five headings do, however, distinguish between broad types of approach involving somewhat different considerations.

The second half of the chapter discusses five common themes in setting up such schemes. In this discussion, we will focus in particular on the voluntary sector, though noting that many of the lessons referred to here apply as much to innovation within the statutory sector:

- Needs, goals and strategies

- Resources

- Recruiting and retaining paid staff and volunteers

- Identifying, stimulating and maintaining demand from carers

- Management issues

Neighbourhood care, community care and sitting schemes

Neighbourhood care is the most general, and perhaps most nebulous, form of support. The strengths and weaknesses of support from 'natural' networks of friends and neighbours have been discussed in Chapter Two. Here the focus is on neighbourhood care *schemes*. Such schemes do various things but in general they aim to provide the sort of support which might ideally be provided by good neighbours. Community care is a notoriously elastic term and may cover a wide range of activities; it refers here to support which is more organised than most neighbourhood care but less intensive than, for example, flexible care attendance. Sitting schemes are self-explanatory and form one part of neighbourhood and community care schemes. What unites these forms of support is that in different ways they aim to galvanise and formalise the types of support caring neighbours might provide.

Before discussing such schemes, some general points need to be made about people's attitudes to giving and receiving support. These points, drawn from the studies of neighbourhood care by Abrams, are fundamental in understanding the contemporary context in which innovations in support for carers recruit and retain helpers and persuade carers to accept support (Abrams *et al.*, 1977, 1980; Bulmer, 1986).

Somewhat depressingly for planners and scheme organisers, the data on attitudes to receiving such care suggest that help from a scheme is not a natural first or even second thought for most people; this suggests that schemes have a long uphill battle to inform users of their existence and to persuade them to accept help. More optimistically the data on attitudes to neighbourhood care also suggest that there is a pool of neighbourhood goodwill which may be tapped, if schemes provide the framework for people to be put in touch with one another. However, it is also suggested that providing a framework for contact and caring is often more difficult than providing direct help, more time-consuming, more expensive and, perhaps, generating fewer measurable results.

On the basis of empirical study of the range of care schemes, three broad types of care can be distinguished. The first is: 'care as working class community'. This type of care needs to be activated by an appropriate organisation – such as a social services department – and those involved will need to be paid. The second type of care is 'care as doing good'. In this type helpers typically do not see themselves as similar to those helped, but wish to establish for themselves a useful and responsible function by doing good to or for others. The third pattern of caring, 'care as trouble shared', is one in which 'helpers are keenly aware of helping as a matter of doing things for one another' arising from 'a need to be freed from the loneliness which they experienced as the normal condition of life before the creation of the neighbourhood group'. (Abrams *et al.*, 1986, p. 67)

Perhaps the single most important message of Abrams' work is that policy makers and practitioners:

> are not left free simply to choose the pattern they happen to prefer. The task rather is to work out which pattern of caring will deliver most care in the light of the social conditions and organisational resources actually available in any given neighbourhood. But that in turn involves understanding the very different social situations and different caring projects (Abrams *et al.*, 1986, p. 67).

Contrary to popular belief, the need for neighbourhood care schemes may be greatest in semi- and un-skilled working-class areas, but these may also be the areas in which schemes are most difficult to organise, especially if helpers are unpaid.

Visiting is considered by most people an acceptable activity for schemes but a wider range of activities might be more acceptable, especially to working-class recipients, if helpers were paid. Reluctance to accept help from unpaid volunteers is emphasised in studies of other types of provision (Moore and Green, 1985; Qureshi *et al.*, 1989; Horton and Berthoud, 1990).

Abrams and his colleagues emphasise that what is provided must be related not only to what people find acceptable and to their needs, but also to the time and long-term continuity helpers are able or willing to provide. Unpaid helpers appear to be able to give only very limited amounts of time per week, whereas paid helpers are able to give more.

Unpaid helpers are most likely to be recruited from among middle-class women not in paid employment, with limited family commitments, belonging to voluntary organisations and with broad religious ideals but not necessarily members of a religious body. But recruiting all helpers (paid or unpaid) is a matter of providing incentives and reducing obstacles to involvement. Payment is one means of increasing the incentive and reducing the obstacles to involvement for working-class women helpers (Qureshi *et al.*, 1987; Leat, 1990). As Abrams and his colleagues point out, the voluntary service model of neighbourhood care presupposes unpaid volunteers and voluntary sector origination and organisation, and may simply be inappropriate for large parts of Britain.

One final point of particular relevance in considering support for carers is worth noting from Abrams' work. Abrams noted that schemes might do more to support carers rather than concentrating their efforts on those cared-for, but the research also highlighted the fact that helpers', and others', perceptions of need were relatively narrow and had moral overtones. It may be more difficult to persuade helpers of the need to enable carers to go shopping or to go away on holiday or to put their feet up than to persuade them of the need to do the shopping for an elderly person living alone.

The Kent Community Care Scheme and its replicas should not be seen primarily as exercises in neighbourhood care – they are, as has been discussed in Chapter Three, concerned with wider organisational and management issues. But such schemes draw and build upon notions of what neighbours might be prepared to do. Evaluation of the Kent scheme highlights the importance of reciprocity in helping – helpers need to get something out of caring if they are to stay involved – a point already made by Abrams. Payment is one means of 'balancing the relationship', from the viewpoint of helpers and users, but payment alone is not enough. Helpers also need continuing support and carefully constructed boundaries to their involvement if they are not to become overloaded and drop out (Qureshi *et al.*, 1989). The evaluation of the scheme illustrates the potential role of social workers as middlemen between users and helpers, but the way in which this operates raises questions about the management of helpers by workers whose first commitment is to the user and to their department. This issue has important implications for arrangements under contracting.

Sitting services can be part of what neighbourhood and community care schemes offer, or a 'fragmentary' service offered in isolation or in relation to the assumed availability of other services. In a sense, sitting services are a re-orientation of the much older voluntary visiting services intended to provide companionship or to reduce isolation for dependent people. Although similar to visiting schemes in many respects, it is obviously crucial that schemes are clear whether the goal is support for carers or companionship for socially isolated people. These goals imply different allocation criteria, organisation and demands on the time of helpers – one hour per day may be enough to reduce social isolation but of little help in enabling carers to take a break or to get out.

Sitting services can experience many of the problems discussed above. Volunteers may not easily or immediately recognise the needs of carers, and some may find 'just sitting' more difficult than performing some practical task. In addition volunteers may find sitting with, for example, demented elderly people very demanding (May *et al.*, 1986). Other difficulties include identifying carers; professionals' reluctance to refer; and the inflexible and somewhat limited nature of the organisation and its resources including the amount and timing of volunteer help.

The impact of sitting services on carers is not entirely clear. Thornton reported many favourable comments in her interviews with recipients (Thornton, 1989). However there are questions to be raised concerning the limited relevance to carers of a service which they may receive for only a few hours per month – if that – and at fixed or limited times. Some carers may see volunteer sitters as an implicit criticism of their own commitment (May *et al.*, 1986). Carers may also be reluctant to use sitting services if they perceive these as receiving 'charity', if they are reluctant to impose on unpaid volunteers, if they are not confident of the helper's ability to cope or of his/her reliability or acceptance of the cared-for person (Moore and Green, 1985). It is possible that payment of sitters may overcome some of these problems (see below).

To summarise:

- Help from a voluntary scheme is not a natural first or even second thought for most people.

- Payment of helpers may make help more acceptable, and increase the range of help considered acceptable and the availability of helpers, especially in working class areas where support may be most needed.

- Helpers need continuing support and carefully constructed boundaries to their involvement if they are not to become overloaded and drop out.

Flexible care attendance

Flexible care attendance is distinguished from neighbourhood care and sitting services insofar as it typically provides more intensive help often on a more regular, if in some cases, infrequent, basis. Various studies suggest that carers value such schemes (Twigg *et al.*, 1990). Factors associated with satisfaction are: the flexibility, regularity and reliability of help; the degree of control carers can exercise over what is provided and by whom; and whether or not the helper is paid. Schemes providing domiciliary help for carers and those they care for have been initiated by social services departments, health authorities, voluntary organisations and, after a slow start, by the private sector.

Some of the best-known and most successful schemes providing domiciliary help specifically for carers are those run by Crossroads care attendants. The first Crossroads scheme was established in 1974 to provide:

Care attendants to relieve the carers of severely physically disabled people. The care attendants ... come at the time when the carers most need the relief, to act as a substitute for the carers to enable the carers to do whatever they need or want to do. Whilst in the home, the care attendant carried out whatever tasks would normally be done by the carer (Bristow, 1981 p. 7).

Significantly, attendants regard themselves as a support to and under the 'direction' of carers rather than those they care for. The most frequently mentioned benefits of such schemes are freedom for the carer (52 per cent), peace of mind (39 per cent) and relief from physical and emotional strain (26 per cent each) (Bristow, 1986). Crossroads Care Attendant schemes have grown rapidly, and by 1991 there were 183 schemes providing one and a half million care hours to 15,000 families. The tasks undertaken by attendants are varied and include getting the disabled person up and dressed in the morning, regular visits during the day when the carer is out, providing occasional holiday or weekend breaks, help with toileting, bathing, meals and so on, as well as overnight stays. Care attendants are not meant to replace statutory services and their help is very clearly and specifically focused on relieving carers rather than the cared-for person.

Unlike many helpers, Crossroads attendants are paid at 'the market rate' tied to local authority scales and are employees rather than freelance workers, employed by the scheme with direct and clear lines of accountability to scheme organisers and ultimately to the management committee. However, in most schemes attendants are paid only for those (flexible) hours they work rather than a weekly or monthly salary. Until now schemes have been funded by a mixture of local authority grants, grants from trusts and local fundraising. The total hours they are able to provide is limited largely by the funds available to pay attendants. Crossroads do not typically charge users for the service and there is considerable resistance to doing so. Dependence on statutory and voluntary funding necessarily limits the total number of care hours a scheme can provide and waiting lists in many areas are long. In the future, schemes are likely to be funded under contractual agreements with local or health authorities rather than grants and there is anxiety that charging carers will become more common.

Issues of funding, charging and costing are central to the current and future operation of schemes. Crossroads emphasise the importance of management, co-ordination, training and, in particular, support for helpers but these entail costs which must be built into estimates of cost per care hour provided. For these reasons the cost of one Crossroads hour may appear high in comparison with schemes providing less management, co-ordination, training and support to helpers. Part of the cost of the flexible care provided by Crossroads is, in a sense, borne by the attendants in the form of uncertain hours and uncertain income; there is some evidence that this uncertainty can lead to drop out and loss of continuity of care for the carer. Attendants paid a salary may stay longer but this obviously increases costs of the scheme (Hopper and Roberts, undated).

Crossroads are increasingly involved in providing attendants to persons in receipt of Independent Living Fund (ILF) monies. The ILF model of provision is quite different from all other approaches considered here insofar as it puts money directly into the hands of disabled people in order that they may purchase whatever help they consider appropriate. ILF funds are not designed to relieve carers but to promote independent living – in doing the latter they may, of course, achieve the former. Research to date has not explored the effects on carers of ILF monies (Kestenbaum, 1990); giving money directly to the dependent person may bypass the carer's needs and preferences, change the relationship between carer and cared-for and introduce a new, and perhaps more difficult, role and responsibility for the carer.

The involvement of schemes in supplying attendants paid for by disabled people out of ILF funds raises important issues of relevance to any organisation or scheme currently involved in or considering such involvement. Providing help to disabled people raises issues about Crossroads' commitment to serving the interests of the carer, about its carefully protected right to retain control over assessment of need, about charging and about the management and accountability of the attendant.

To summarise:

- Carers value the support of care assistants. The factors associated with satisfaction are: the regularity of help; the degree of control carers can exercise over what is provided and by whom; and whether or not the helper is paid.

- Dependence on statutory and voluntary funding limits the total number of care hours schemes can provide; and waiting lists in many areas are long.

- Schemes need to consider the management, co-ordination, training and, in particular, support for helpers but these entail costs which must be built into estimates of cost per care hour provided.

Flexible Respite
A broad distinction can be drawn here between family-based respite care which is largely provided for children with learning disabilities and other forms of flexible home-based respite. The distinction is somewhat arbitrary; and the success of family-based schemes for children, which now represent the preferred form of respite support, has clearly provided models for the development of services for other client groups.

Family-based respite care schemes largely cater for children with learning disabilities and, to an extent, adults. Their attitude to carers is slightly ambiguous – relief for carers is stressed but so too is 'normalisation' and the right of all to family rather than institutional care. Emphasis on the needs of the disabled child seems to have grown in recent years, at the expense of an emphasis on supporting the carers, although in many cases the two will be indistinguishable.

Family-based respite care schemes have grown rapidly in recent years. At the end of the 1970s 16 schemes were in operation rising to over 265 schemes by 1991; all but 53 of these 265 schemes were for children (Orlik et al., 1991). Many schemes provided a range of help including befriending, and home care, as well as respite care in the helper's home. Helpers are typically semi-paid (that is, paid at a rate which is not presented as being the market rate) although some are fully paid and some, mainly those involved in befriending, receive no payment. Rates of pay vary dramatically from scheme to scheme and appear to bear no relation to what is being requested of helpers. Most schemes pay helpers on a sessional basis which is presumably administratively easier for organisers, families and helpers than 'clock- watching' on an hourly rate. A small number of schemes pay retainers in addition to sessional fees. Interestingly, Orklik et al. suggest that: 'Retainer paid carers are not a popular option since they tend to be linked to a lot of different children. Problems therefore may arise around availability' (Orlik et al., 1991, p.10).

Evidence suggests that those carers who receive the service find it helpful. But it should be noted that the majority of schemes provide care for children only, so that as carers themselves become older less rather than more help is likely to be available. Around half of all schemes provide help totalling less than six weeks per person, per annum, often allocated on a voucher system. Just over one-third of schemes say that there is no limit to the amount of respite care which can be provided. Operating with no limit on the care available may only be feasible because parents' 'own desire to provide care coupled with their feelings of guilt tend to act as a barrier to seeking additional respite for their children'. Parents need encouragement to take up respite care:

> 'One wonders how co-ordinators could manage their budgets if parents on the fifty schemes offering unlimited care did actually increase their use of service.' (Orlik et al., 1991, p. 17).

The majority of schemes have a waiting list; and insofar as some part of the waiting list is composed of those people with challenging behaviour and severe physical disabilities whom many schemes find the most difficult to place, some carers may have a longer wait than others. Men are also harder to place, possibly because most helpers are women and prefer to care for other women; men with challenging behaviour may also pose particular problems. Further difficulties may arise in placing people from ethnic minorities; and the number of ethnic minority users exceeds that of helpers. The most effective method of recruiting both users and helpers from ethnic minorities is to employ ethnic minorities staff.

Waiting lists may also be attributed to a shortage of helpers, but on closer inspection this shortage, especially for adult schemes, seems to come down to the fact that adult schemes have lower budgets, fewer staff hours and pay their helpers less; potential helpers are available but there are not enough staff to recruit them.

Not all flexible respite is provided on this family model. As noted at the start of this section, there are other forms of flexible home-based respite. These are mainly provided for older people and can take a variety of forms. For example, the Age Concern scheme described by Thornton (1989) provides a mixture of help, ranging from respite in the helper's home, live-in respite in the home of the older person or his or her carer, as well as a variety of forms of day care. In general the emphasis in these schemes is on relief for the carer, though they can also be used to give an older or disabled person a break from his or her home. The 'family' ideology that dominates schemes for children and young people with learning disabilities is also less marked. In the late 1970s there were estimated to be 23 such schemes: by 1990 this had risen to at least 170 (Thornton and Moore, 1960; BASW, 1991). Much of the growth in adult family placement occurred on the basis of the availability of residential care benefits to pay for such care, thus giving local authorities an incentive to develop such schemes (Todd and Young, 1988; Young, 1988).

The limited evidence available on carer satisfaction with such schemes suggests that once persuaded to use them, carers value the break they provide (Leat, 1983; SSI,1990). Although the majority of care is provided in the helper's home, more recently some schemes have been experimenting with respite care in the user's home. Care provided in the user's home may minimise the disruption and confusion for the user and may be what carers prefer (Hills, 1991). But it may be more difficult to recruit helpers who are able or prepared to spend time away from their own homes (Thornton, 1989; Hills, 1991). Furthermore, it may be argued that such an arrangement does not give the carer the option of staying at home and fails to provide the cared-for with the stimulation of a change of scenery.

Unlike Crossroads attendants, these helpers are not typically paid an hourly rate related to the market rate but are paid highly variable amounts often related to the benefits which can be pieced together for each individual user, or on a standard, very low hourly or sessional rate which is most often presented as a token payment rather than any real reflection of the value of what is done.

Management costs are usually covered by the local authority or voluntary organisation running the scheme and in some cases, especially since changes in the availability of benefits, some payments to helpers are also wholly provided or are 'topped-up' from such sources.

The difficulties faced by adult family placement schemes are similar to those already outlined. Schemes are not widely known amongst potential users and they must overcome problems related to public acceptability and confidence as well as carers' guilt about leaving the cared-for person (Leat, 1983; SSI,1990; Orlik et al., 1990; Thornton, 1989). When older helpers are employed or if the level of pay is very low, users may be additionally reluctant to 'impose' on helpers (Thornton, 1989). Professionals also may not understand the scope or potential of schemes, may be reluctant to refer to the scheme or may query the level of client dependency appropriate to schemes. 'Solving' the problem of referrals by encouraging self-referral may create difficulties in targeting.

At present many schemes are poorly co-ordinated with other types of service provision. This may partly be due to their lack of integration within social services departments and health authorities which in turn is related to their early dependence on social security benefits.

Schemes currently appear to have little difficulty in recruiting suitable helpers, although there may be greater difficulty in finding helpers willing to spend time away from home. Lack of helpers with suitable accommodation may be a problem in some areas; helpers obviously need the space to accommodate an extra person and in some cases may need ground floor facilities or aids and adaptations. Recruitment of helpers may be increasingly affected by social security funding regulations which act as a deterrent to one-helper households and those dependent on state benefits and lower incomes. Various studies have noted that the level of remuneration to helpers varies dramatically and appears to bear little relation to the demands made (Leat and Gay, 1987; SSI, 1990). Although there is no evidence that helpers become involved solely, or even mainly, for the money, the perceived adequacy of the level of pay may change over time (Qureshi et al., 1987, Leat, 1990). If helpers are to be retained, regular reviews of payments should be conducted related to both rises in the cost of living and the circumstances of users and helpers. Scheme co-ordinators may also need to spend time advising users on sources of funding or benefits to pay for care, and helpers on the tax and benefit implications of being paid. Insurance and legal protection for users and helpers also require attention.

Some schemes experience difficulties in balancing the supply of helpers with demand. This is not simply a matter of numbers of referrals but equally importantly one of the right helpers available at the right time. Schemes attach great significance to careful matching of helpers and users and there is evidence that users value personal relationships and continuity of help. But without an oversupply of helpers it is likely that choice and continuity will be limited for some users at some times; if helpers have different levels of skill and 'tolerance' for certain types of user, or are not available for, say, live-in care, choice is likely to be further reduced and some helpers may be overused and overloaded. As already noted, the danger of maintaining a sufficient oversupply of helpers to ensure choice for users is that helpers drop out because of underuse.

To summarise:

- Once persuaded to use schemes, carers value the break they provide.

- It may be more difficult to recruit helpers who are able or prepared to spend time away from their own homes.

- Schemes are not widely known amongst potential users, and they must overcome problems related to public and professional acceptability and confidence as well as carers' guilt about leaving the cared-for person.

- If helpers are to be retained, regular reviews of payments should be conducted.

- Some schemes experience difficulties in balancing the supply of helpers with demand from carers.

Information, advice and support

Despite the fact that research has demonstrated that among the priority needs of carers are those of information and emotional support, there has been little evaluation of projects aimed at meeting these needs. This section therefore relies on somewhat sparse data.

In an important sense, providing information to carers should be everyone's business, and there are obvious dangers in separating off information provision as someone else's responsibility. But various projects have attempted to increase the supply and quality of information available to known carers and, most importantly, those 'hidden' carers who are not already in touch with services. Information may range from that concerned with benefits and financial advice to availability of services and sources of help. The timing of information is crucial – it is no good discovering that you could have received x or y when you are no longer eligible or the help is no longer appropriate. Information must also be backed up by available services. Otherwise carers are disappointed, and providing information may be seen as a low-cost, token response with little substance.

Many of the problems in communicating with carers are common to all projects, especially new ones. It is worth noting here, however, that information projects take time to get going and need adequate funding; funding may be particularly difficult to obtain for projects which appear to produce little tangible effect other than to increase demand on other services. Some information providers may be seen as somewhat threatening, especially if they encourage carers to be more demanding, and for that reason may be viewed with some suspicion by professionals (Haffenden, 1991).

Haffenden sums up the essential conditions for providing information to carers. It must be given at the right time and come from a trusted and acceptable source. Information should cover benefits, services and the condition of the cared-for person. Carers should be given help to use the information, and it must be given in simple language and reinforced constantly (Haffenden, 1991).

Although providing information is everyone's job, this may create problems in overlap, specialisation, fragmentation and lack of co-ordination. For many professionals and carers a 'one-stop' carers' centre providing information on a range of issues is likely to be particularly welcome (Haffenden, 1991).

Carers' centres are designed to provide user-friendly specialist information for carers, to co-ordinate information, to provide advocacy for individual carers and generally to raise awareness of carers' needs and ideas for service modifications. The centres studied by Hills and Haffenden as part of their evaluation of the Department of Health's demonstration districts were most likely to reach people early on in their caring 'careers'; primarily used by carers of less dependent people, they may be able to play a key role in identifying carers and helping them sort out problems before a crisis develops. Advocacy was played down because the centres wanted referrals from professionals and did not wish to appear as a threat. Centres can have difficulty is finding funding, partly because they cross-cut funders' priorities and responsibilities, and partly because they provide few tangible results (Hills, 1991).

Despite their relatively high costs, after two years the centres were only reaching a small proportion of carers, suggesting that a longer period of funding is required for maximum effectiveness (Haffenden, 1991).

Apart from providing information' carers' centres are one means of providing emotional support to carers, and those studied by Haffenden were primarily valued for this function. Emotional support may also be provided by carer groups as outlined in Chapter Three. Professional counselling does not seem to be valued by carers, especially is it is provided out of the home and involves making appointments (Haffenden, 1991). Any form of out-of-home support requires a sitting service and transport for carers. Telephone advice and support lines have been shown to be valuable, but they need access to a data base, material to send to callers and to be able to offer face-to-face contact – and all of these features are costly. In addition, helplines need active promotion, and money and time for publicity. Ideally they should be able to provide a service seven days a week (Haffenden, 1991).

Support is often especially valued if it is provided by other carers who understand what it is really like to be a carer. But it is important to note that projects run by carers, or heavily dependent upon carer involvement, are likely to experience special difficulties which in some cases may jeopardise the survival of the scheme (Haffenden, 1991; Hills, 1991).

To summarise:

- Information projects take time to get going and need adequate funding. Funding may be particularly difficult to obtain for projects which appear to produce little tangible effect other than to increase demands on other services.

- Information must be given at the right time and come from a trusted and acceptable source. Carers should be given help to use the information and it must be given in simple language and reinforced constantly.

Consultation and involvement in planning

Sir Roy Griffiths would have been very unlikely to introduce a radical re-structuring of Sainsbury's retailing practices without systematic consumer research in order to ensure that the changes would not drive his erstwhile customers to Tesco or Gateway. No such systematic market research has been conducted with the users of our community care services in advance of the radical overhaul of arrangements for their provision (Jowell, 1991 p. 80).

Schemes which consult and involve carers are not a separate category; consultation and involvement should underpin all schemes designed to support carers. However, there have been a small number of projects in recent years which have been specifically designed to consult carers and involve them in the planning of services. In addition, the advocacy role of organisations such as Carers National Association, MENCAP, MIND and National Schizophrenia Fellowship, among others, has grown. The views of such organisations have been increasingly difficult for policy makers and planners to ignore; and such groups have become involved in consultation and planning at national, and some local, levels. In many spheres the consultation and involvement of users in planning is more rhetoric than reality. There are also important questions to be asked about the extent to which any group should be able to influence political decisions about priorities and the allocation of scarce resources by elected and supposedly representative policy makers. In the provision of support for carers there is also a need to recognise the potential conflict between the interests and needs of carers and those they care for.

In theory at least, the consultation of carers and recognition of their needs and preferences, as distinct from those they care for, is set to increase under the provisions of the 1990 NHS and Community Care Act. The guidance on implementation of the act states that individual care plans should be the result of a 'constructive dialogue between user, carer and social services staff' (DH, 1990). Emphasising 'client-led' services, the objective of the new structure is to involve users and carers more, placing them at the centre of the concerns of agencies, establishing a greater sense of partnership with them in determining the services appropriate to their needs. What this will mean in practice is still unclear. Some argue that the growth of contracting out will, by its very process, increase the ability of voluntary organisations who are providing services to influence the shape and content of provision. Others suggest that the process will do nothing to address the fundamental problem of the rationing and distribution of scarce resources, and as voluntary organisations are drawn into being providers their advocacy role will decrease. From the viewpoint of carers, contracting out to voluntary organisations may mean no more in practice than the replacement of one rationing bureaucracy by another.

One of the best documented projects designed to consult and involve users in planning services has been the Birmingham Community Care Special Action Project. The project's brief was:

> To develop corporate approaches to community care, thereby harnessing resources beyond just the health and social services partnership; to utilise the expertise of service users and their carers in guiding the planning and development of services; and ensure that in the light of the corporate user-led objectives the City Council was making the best use of existing resources.

Two points are particularly important. First, the project was not seen as a discrete initiative but as a vehicle for change across the whole city, permeating all planning in relation to community care provision. Secondly, the emphasis was on: 'the achievement of short-term service improvements substantially within existing resources'; and on finding innovative approaches to meet service users' requirements (including those from ethnic minorities). None of these requirements had major resource implications. The project employed a variety of methods including consultations with carers at public meetings. These consultations involved extensive publicity, the provision of transport and refreshments and alternative care arrangements to enable carers to attend. Professionals were allowed to attend, but were not allowed to contribute. Users' views were then translated into plans which were tested through a programme of limited small-scale local pilots.

On the basis of the project's experience Jowell identified four major requirement of any such programme:

- There must be corporate processes to guide user-led community care which fit existing committee processes and are capable of being monitored and influenced by members; political support and commitment are essential.

- There must be chief officer commitment and executive authority to ensure the implementation of new ideas.

- There must be space, an acceptance of risk-taking and innovation and support for fresh ways of thinking.

- User-led approaches must be embedded in a new service culture by, for example, including user-responsiveness as a performance target in the contract of chief officers (Jowell, 1991).

Consultation on this scale is certainly neither quick nor easy nor cheap; and the requirements listed above are no mean agenda for any organisation. But the effects of consultation may pay dividends in more efficient use of resources and better quality, more relevant services. Consultation with carers does not, of course, have to be on the scale of the Birmingham project but token gestures undertaken without careful planning, clearly specified limits (for example, are extra resources available?) and feed-back to carers are unlikely to achieve much, and may be positively damaging (Haffenden, 1991; on other methods of consultation see also Richardson et al., 1989).

To summarise:

- There must be genuine political and executive commitment to user-led planning.

- Token gestures undertaken without careful planning, clearly specified limits and feed-back to carers are unlikely to achieve much and may be positively damaging.

Common themes in innovation

Some problems in developing new services or approaches are peculiar to particular types of provision or ways of working, but what is striking about the literature on innovation is the way in which com-

mon themes recur. Five common themes are discussed below, drawing attention to similarities and differences arising in particular
types of innovation. This discussion will concentrate largely on the
particular issues posed by innovation within the voluntary sector.

Needs, goals and strategies

The notion that innovative businesses are those which are constantly in touch with their customers is now widely accepted (Peters and
Austin, 1985). Identifying users' needs and preferences is no less
important in non-profit voluntary and statutory organisations. Thus
the first step in developing new provision for carers is to *identify
what carers want*.

The needs and preferences of carers, and the differences between
carers, have been discussed above in Chapter Two but the importance of starting from what (different) carers want bears repetition.
Various studies have shown that research into carers' real needs,
and consultation with carers, pays off in more successful provision
(Haffenden, 1991).

As emphasised above, the needs and preferences of carers vary,
and for that reason it is essential to be clear about precisely *which
groups of carers, with what needs, the intended project is designed to help*.
The needs of ethnic minority carers, for example, will certainly
require special methods of publicity and of provision.

Having identified a key target group and their needs, it is also
important to consider *what other services are available*. Those involved
in the development of new services – especially in the voluntary sector – have an understandable tendency to see a need and then set
about meeting it without always considering how this might be integrated or co-ordinated with other services (Moore and Green, 1985).
The danger of this approach is that the project or service is less than
fully effective or is an isolated 'fragment' rather than part of a wider
package of provision which is as a whole more relevant to carers
than the sum of its parts. Lack of consideration of the availability of
other services may be not merely less than fully effective from the
viewpoint of carers, but may actually damage the achievement of
the project's goals:

> 'A sitting service without the information service that re-
> ferred the carer or the support group that enabled the carer to
> cope with the guilt engendered by using the service may have
> made little difference' (Hodgson and Hills, quoted in Hills, 1991
> p. 78).

Consideration of the availability of other services may lead to the
need to consider offering something more than or different from the
service originally envisaged, or it may mean attempting to

coordinate better or re-mix existing services rather than developing anything new.

Identifying a target group, and assessing the availability of other services are the essential background to *formulation of clear and realistic goals and strategies*. One reason why projects fail is a lack of clear goals (Hills, 1991; Haffenden, 1991). But goals, and strategies to achieve those goals, must also be realistic. One of the strongest messages from the literature on innovation in this field is that everything takes longer than anticipated and that the scope and scale of new projects that survive tend to be small (Moore and Green, 1985; Hadley *et al.*, 1984; Haffenden, 1991; Hills, 1991). Realistic – small-scale and 'slow' – goals not only reduce the risk of failure by refusing to set over-ambitious, unachievable standards but also avoid the dangers of 'organisational overload' which is another cause of failure in new ventures in support for carers or of other groups (Hills, 1991).

Strategies must obviously be linked to goals, but devising appropriate and workable strategies also requires *recognition of the conditions and constraints* on service development and use by carers. Constraints on service development vary in relation to what is being provided, how and by whom, and some of these are discussed below. But there are also some more fundamental constraints which must be considered in all types of provision.

Among these are the character and culture of the area. Developments for carers in rural areas with scattered populations, lack of public transport and typically small, less formally organised voluntary organisations are likely to require more time and more resources in money and time from development staff. Without adequate time, resources and professional input, it may be more realistic to consider carefully the scope for piecing together services for carers rather than starting anything new (Haffenden, 1991). In urban areas populations of carers may be more concentrated but also more diverse; transport may be better; and voluntary organisations less 'fragile' and better able to take on board new work.

The culture of an area may also create constraints on organisation. For example, in working-class areas, with no tradition of volunteering and few women with the time and freedom from domestic and economic demands, it may be more difficult to recruit unpaid volunteers (Abrams *et al.*, 1986). In close-knit urban and rural areas carers may be reluctant to use certain types of service provided by friends and neighbours especially if these involve sharing private information, for example about money. Similarly, developments for ethnic minority carers may face particular constraints on the type of helpers considered acceptable (for example, the same sex, race or religion) and further difficulties in attracting both helpers and users (Orlik *et al.*, 1991).

This section has stressed the importance of having clear target groups, clear identification of needs and preferences, clear and realistic goals, and carefully considered strategies constructed in the light of constraints on both provision and use. However, despite the very best preparation, a project may find that it has missed a sometimes small but crucial point and it should have the flexibility to adapt its operation accordingly; in day care, for example, carers may be grateful for Saturday afternoon off but may prefer Saturday morning to do the shopping or Sunday afternoon to relax or to be with other members of the family, or vice versa. The need for flexibility also arises from the simple fact that carers' needs change, and the project may need to change accordingly. Some of the difficulties in combining clarity in goals and strategies with flexibility in practice are discussed in more detail below.

To summarise:

- The aims of a project need to be considered in the context of what other services are available locally.

- The character and culture of the area affects what can be provided.

- One reason why projects fail is lack of clear goals.

- Everything takes longer than anticipated; the scope and scale of new projects which survive tend to be small.

Resources
All developments require resources – time, money and labour – which must be borne by someone, whether central or local government, charities, existing staff or volunteers. Clearly, the availability of money, time and labour are interrelated – money can buy time and labour but conversely time and labour may be required to obtain money. The need for time to do background research, to plan, to set up the project, to get it going and to keep it going is a recurring theme in studies of innovation for carers, and all of these are likely to take longer than originally anticipated.

Different types of provision are likely to require more money, time and labour than others depending on what is being provided, for whom, for how many, by whom, how and where. Even if nothing new is being provided and the innovations are a matter of making better use of existing services or better co-ordination there will still be resource implications. Using existing staff to develop new ways of working will at the least entail opportunity costs in staff time; such an approach may be particularly vulnerable to disruption by the demands of existing work, staff absence and turn-over (Hadley *et al.*, 1984; Orlik *et al.*, 1991).

Costs do, however, vary between types of provision. These costs may be more or less visible and may or may not be borne by those initiating the service. So, for example, providing respite or day care may be more costly than a sitting service in the carer's home, but the costs for some groups may be recoverable, from charges to the user and/or from benefits. Some of the costs of day care may be 'hidden' in the provision of free accommodation, lighting, heating and so on. Developing services for 'invisible' carers not already in touch with professionals, or for ethnic minority carers, are likely to be more costly because they are harder to reach; require more and different publicity; need more helpers or more or specially recruited staff; and will take longer to get going (Orlik et al., 1991). Services for carers in rural areas may be more costly in staff time, transport and publicity than those in urban areas and may end up serving fewer people. Services provided by volunteers are not necessarily cheaper than those using paid staff not least because involving volunteers will require more publicity, more organisation, greater support and may serve those who are less dependent (Haffenden, 1991). The use of volunteers is discussed in more detail below.

In planning any development it is essential to consider all costs (money, time and labour) above and below the line, and to identify clearly the total cost and likely sources of funding and 'free' resources and over what period these will be required, bearing in mind the emphasis above on the time required to get things going. It is also important to remember that some of the early start-up costs may disappear, only to be replaced by the costs associated with increased demand (Leat, 1983).

One of the difficulties faced by many innovative projects for carers is that they are given only six or twelve months to get going. As a result some projects start only to fail, either because further funding is not available or because valuable staff development time has been spent on the desperate search for further funding. Short-term funding may also inhibit development by preventing longer-term planning. For most developments three to five years' support may be a more realistic, efficient and effective use of money. For many projects the problems of funding do not disappear once they become 'established'; indeed their problems may increase insofar as it is easier to obtain funding from charitable trusts and statutory grant-givers for something new rather than for something which has been tried and tested. Once a project can no longer be presented as 'innovative' it will almost certainly require local or health authority support if it is to survive (Haffenden, 1991). In order to obtain such support a project will need to be able to demonstrate its worth, and for this reason record-keeping, monitoring and evaluation are important aids to survival.

Innovative projects for carers which cut across existing service boundaries and responsibilities may have particular difficulty in obtaining funding for that very reason. This difficulty may be exacerbated if the project also produces few tangible results (Hills, 1991).

Finally, in considering funding bids it is important to bear in mind the points above regarding flexibility. The dilemma for some projects is that a good funding application should be clear about goals, strategies and costs, but too tight an application may constrain the project's subsequent freedom for manoeuvre in responding to carers' changing needs. A related difficulty is that funding must usually be obtained before staff are appointed, but too tight a proposal may create difficulties for staff not involved in the initial application in putting plans into practice (Moore and Green, 1985).

To summarise:

- Developing services for 'invisible' carers not already in touch with professionals or for rural and ethnic minority carers is likely to be more costly and will take longer to get going.

- Services provided by volunteers are not necessarily cheaper than those using paid staff.

- Projects need adequate funding and time to get going; the problems of funding do not disappear once the project becomes 'established'.

- Innovative projects which cut across existing service boundaries and responsibilities may have particular difficulty in obtaining funding.

Recruiting and keeping volunteers and paid staff

To pay or not to pay? Depending on the type of development, reliance on volunteers may or may not be an option. There is some evidence to suggest that volunteers are not necessarily a cheaper option than paid staff and, in any case, few projects for carers can operate efficiently with no paid staff (Leat *et al.*, 1986; Haffenden, 1991). The difficulty in relying substantially on volunteers is that in many areas they are hard to find and may become even harder to find as demand for women to return to the paid labour market increases and as voluntary organisations increasingly become involved in contract work for local authorities. Volunteers typically work for only a few hours per week and it is therefore necessary to have a lot of them to provide a regular service to even a very small number of people. Recruiting large numbers of volunteers, co-ordinating them, training and supporting and keeping them not only requires some paid staff but may also cost more than employing a smaller number of part- or full-time paid staff. Furthermore, some types of development, in rural areas for example, may require skills and longer-term commitment of time not readily available from unpaid volunteers.

The disadvantages of paying volunteers are obviously the cost and, some would argue, the effects on the relationship between helper and user and the danger of attracting people who are 'only in it for the money'. The advantages of paying volunteers are assumed to be increased supply, greater commitment of time and effort, greater reliability, greater control or accountability (Leat and Gay, 1987). In some areas with little tradition of voluntary service and other pressures on women's time, it has been argued that paying volunteers is the only option (Abrams *et al.*, 1986). Another argument in favour of paying volunteers is that this makes help more acceptable to carers and increases the likelihood that they will use the service as and when they need it (Moore and Green, 1985). Given the difficulties in persuading carers to accept help, this last argument may be particularly strong.

One of the most valued characteristics of some innovative projects is their flexibility in providing carers with what they want when they want or need it. The cost of providing an 'on-call' service is, of course, very high and most projects have significantly reduced these costs by involving paid or semi-paid, usually but not always freelance, workers who are paid only for the hours they actually work. The difficulty with this approach is that helpers suffer from insecurity of income and this may be one source of dissatisfaction and ultimately drop-out (Leat, 1990; Hopper and Roberts, undated). Payment of retainers between periods of helping is one solution to this difficulty but is still relatively unusual even in established areas of provision such as child fostering. Payment of a regular wage or salary is another solution, but is likely to reduce flexibility and personal matching and will increase costs – although it may also increase reliability and continuity (Orlik *et al,*. 1991).

Whether or not volunteers are paid for their time or labour, they will almost certainly need expenses and these will obviously vary depending on the nature and location of the help provided. How expenses are paid is important; if expenses are not clearly itemised and paid on the basis of costs actually incurred they are liable to be taxed or deducted from the volunteer's benefit.

Recruitment and retention
When paid staff are employed the greater difficulty may lie not so much in recruiting them as in keeping them, especially if salaries are low or if funding is short-term or insecure. Recruiting volunteers may be more difficult depending on the type of area, the type of work involved, the type of volunteers required and whether or not expenses and payment are offered. There are various avenues through which volunteers may be recruited, including volunteer

bureaux, churches, local community groups and other organisations as well as via local radio, the local press and posters.

Leafleting is time-consuming and labour-intensive and the results may be poor initially. Leaflets may, however, have 'a slow trickle down effect in which the memory of the leaflet stays in people's minds and may be recalled some time later'. Local newspapers may give an opportunity to provide more detailed, illustrative information about the type of volunteers and commitment required than, for example, television advertising which may generate a lot of interest but 'much time is wasted in replying to people who subsequently prove to be unsuitable' (Orlik et al., 1991 p. 24).

Projects vary in the extent to which they engage in rigorous selection procedures for volunteers. In the wake of some recent, well-publicised tragedies and the growth of contracting, asking for and taking up references, at the least, may become more widespread. For work involving children, references and police checks are minimum requirements.

Volunteers not only need to be recruited, selected, matched, introduced and allocated, they also need to be prepared, trained and above all, supported. I shall discuss training and support of volunteers in more detail below.

Volunteers, unpaid and semi-paid, are liable to drop out if too much is expected of them and if too little is asked of them (Qureshi et al., 1987; Abrams et al., 1986). In the early stages of a new development for carers, having too many volunteers and too few carer-users may be the greatest problem but when volunteers start dropping out due to under-use demand may pick up which the project is then unable to meet. Balancing supply and demand, and keeping it balanced, is therefore a continuing problem for most projects.

To summarise:

- The disadvantages of paying volunteers are the cost, and the assumed effects on the relationship between helper and user.

- The advantages are assumed to be increased supply, greater commitment of time and effort, greater reliability, greater control or accountability and greater acceptability to users.

- Recruitment tactics need to match the nature of the area.

- Volunteers are liable to drop out if too little or too much is expected of them.

Identifying, stimulating and maintaining demand from carers

Attracting users is ironically one of the most difficult tasks new projects for carers have to face. Identifying hidden carers not already in

117

touch with services is a problem for both statutory and voluntary organisations. One obvious route to hidden carers is via general practitioners, but despite the efforts of various bodies this may not be an entirely satisfactory method, not least because, as we have noted in Chapter Three, carers may remain 'invisible' to their GPs.

In small community projects with local volunteers and an organiser living locally, it may be possible to identify carers by working through local networks and word of mouth (Moore and Green, 1985). But such methods are necessarily limited in scale and are not appropriate in other areas, although some of the benefits of local knowledge may be obtained by splitting projects up into small geographical units. In most projects however some publicity will be needed to attract carers.

Various methods of publicity are suggested in the literature including posters, information to other organisations and via libraries and CABx, advertisements, local radio features, articles in local papers, exhibitions and travelling road-shows. Obviously one key criterion in the choice of forms of publicity must be where carers go and what they are likely to see or hear. However, seeing or hearing information about provision is not always sufficient because carers do not necessarily recognise themselves as such. For this reason an article in a local newspaper may be more effective than an advertisement because it allows for discussion and illustration of the sort of people the project is aiming to help and the sort of help it can offer. Because carers do not 'self-identify', it is important that information stands are manned by people who understand the project and can talk to people and answer their queries, encouraging them to make contact with the project if appropriate. In general impersonal publicity needs to be reinforced by personal contact (Moore and Green, 1985; Haffenden, 1991).

Information stands should also be located where it is possible to have a conversation without being overheard; for this reason GPs' waiting rooms may not be the best location (Haffenden, 1991). Particular problems arise in projects designed to support ethnic minority carers. Employing ethnic minority staff may be the most effective way of reaching both ethnic minority carers and helpers (Orlik et al., 1991). Finally, of course, publicity is unlikely to be very effective unless carers are followed up and offered, indeed encouraged to use, the services on offer (Moore and Green, 1987).

Reaching known carers is by definition easier for statutory services but may be difficult for voluntary sector projects. Various studies have demonstrated the difficulties faced by voluntary projects, and some new projects in statutory organisations, in getting referrals from professional workers (Leat, 1983; Moore and Green, 1985; Haffenden,1991). Informing professionals of the existence and work of the project is unlikely to produce many, if any, referrals, not east because such information is likely to get 'lost' in the organisation (Moore and Green, 1985). More importantly, however, new projects must find a way of overcoming professionals' worries about and objections to new services for carers, especially those run by volunteers and voluntary organisations. Professionals worry about breaching confidentiality by passing on names of carers, they worry that volunteers as non-professionals may do more harm than good and may be unreliable, raising expectations and then not meeting them. They worry that they do not have sufficient control over provision to be able to offer it to their clients with integrity; and they justify their reluctance to use services in terms of a belief that clients share these worries. They believe that carers prefer professional services and would be unhappy leaving those they care for with an unqualified person. They believe that carers and their dependants do not want strangers in the house; and they suggest that few services can offer the immediate 'now, not next month' help that carers really want and need (Moore and Green, 1985; Leat, 1983). When professionals are persuaded to refer clients to project, they may provide inappropriate referrals (Leat, 1983; Moore and Green, 1985).

The only way around these difficulties seems to be through constant and careful selling of the scheme, preferably by personal contact rather than written information or on the telephone. This will occupy a large part of the organiser's time in the early stages of the project and may at first produce few results. Results are most likely to be achieved as a result of a small number of 'successes' – having worked successfully with a few referrals, more will follow and word will spread (Leat, 1983; Moore and Green, 1985). The problem for new ventures is therefore to break through that initial barrier, to establish a track record on which trust can be built and grow. Having had a few 'satisfied customers' a project needs to use these to inspire further confidence and trust.

Identifying carers is only a first step in stimulating demand – carers must also be persuaded to use the service and that too may not be easy. Carers may be reluctant to use the service because they do not see it as being for them; because they do not want to accept 'charity' or are worried about 'imposing' on, especially, older helpers; because they are reluctant to take a break at all, or because they are unhappy about leaving the cared-for person with a stranger or with a non-professional (Leat, 1983; Moore and Green, 1987; Orlik et al., 1991; Thornton, 1989). The barriers to be overcome will vary between carers and in relation to the type of service being offered.

Assuming that the project is offering something relevant to the particular carer, the major difficulty is likely to be one of establishing trust and, in some cases, of overcoming guilt about admitting to wanting or needing a break and about leaving the cared-for person. Establishing trust with the carer and the cared-for person is likely to

119

be a slow process and will almost certainly require several visits (Flynn, 1989). Again, carers are likely to be encouraged by hearing of others who have used the project satisfactorily, and the process of establishing trust may become easier as the project acquires satisfied customers to whom it can refer prospective users. Although carers may find a service focused on their needs more helpful than one designed for the benefit of the person they care for, there is also some evidence to suggest that presentation of the service in terms of benefit to the cared-for person may lead to greater take-up than presentation in terms of relief for the carer (Moore and Green, 1985). Maintaining the demand from carers and the supply of helpers is likely to depend partly on how they experience their relationship with each other. Careful matching of carers and helpers may be one means of encouraging a satisfactory relationship for both parties.

The importance attached to careful matching varies between projects depending in part on the type of service being offered. For some types of intensive care and for some groups of carers, a degree of matching is likely to be essential; for example, services for ethnic minorities need to practise careful matching and so may those providing respite care. In reality, however, especially in emergency situations or when there is less than an over-supply of volunteers, matching may have to be crude, if it is possible at all. In some types of project, matching may be done on a geographical basis reducing the amount of time spent travelling for volunteers and encouraging informal links between helpers and carers, but in some cases carers may prefer to receive help from those who do not live nearby.

In the early stages of a project when demand is low, carers may be able to have help more or less as often as they wish. But at some stage most projects will need to address the difficult issue of rationing help – of deciding who gets what and how often. The question of who is in control of assessment and allocation is likely to assume greater importance in the context of contracting, and many voluntary organisations will want to retain the right to some degree of control over both. Some respite care projects, for example, adopt a voucher system where, having been assessed as qualifying for help, carers are provided with vouchers which entitle them to x hours of help per month or per year. This system has the advantage of allowing the project overall control over allocation of resources, but at the same time gives carers a relatively high degree of flexibility and control over when they use that help. Vouchers may also reduce the administrative costs of a project because arrangements are left to carers and helpers but, at the same time, they may increase costs for volunteers who cannot plan their involvement and who do not receive payment at the time of placement. It may also increase costs to the project which cannot make maximum efficient use of the workforce available.

Volunteers not only need to be recruited, selected, matched, introduced and allocated, they also need to be prepared/trained and, above all, supported. I shall discuss training and support of volunteers in more detail below. At this point it is important to note that providing support for carers and involving and supporting volunteers are intimately related. Every project involving volunteers needs to aim to achieve a constant balance between supply and demand. Too few volunteers, or too many or too few inadequately managed volunteers, will mean an inadequate and unreliable service for carers or volunteer overload and drop-out; too many volunteers will lead to under use, drop-out and possibly a future shortage of volunteers just when the service is expanding and they are most needed.

To summarise:

- Attracting users is one of the most difficult tasks new projects for carers have to face.

- Seeing or hearing information about provision is not sufficient because carers do not necessarily identify themselves as such. Publicity should include discussion and illustration of the sort of people the project is aiming to help and the sort of help it can offer.

- Publicity is unlikely to be effective unless carers are followed up and offered, indeed encouraged, to use the services on offer.

- Establishing trust with the carer and the cared-for person is likely to be a slow process and will almost certainly require several visits.

- New projects must find a way of overcoming professionals' worries about and objections to new services for carers by constant and careful selling of the scheme, preferably by personal contact rather than written information or on the telephone.

- At some stage most projects will need to address the difficult issue of rationing help.

Management issues

The need for clear goals and strategies, realistic costings and timetables has already been emphasised. The need for flexibility built into project goals and strategies – the aim to provide a flexible service, for example – as well as a degree of flexibility in the definition of goals was also stressed. Achieving this balancing act between clarity and flexibility is likely to be difficult and may be achieved by what management theorists refer to as 'loose- tight' structures in which certain

121

core values and tasks are very clearly defined, but the ways in which those are pursued is open to adaptation and experiment in the light of changing needs and consumer demands (Peters and Austin, 1985; Handy, 1989).

Managers will also need to ensure that workers are clear about their individual and collective roles and tasks. Confusion and ambiguity in workers' and volunteers' roles and tasks has been identified as one cause of failure in new projects (Haffenden, 1991). Clarity in roles, tasks and commitments may be especially important in voluntary organisations and in projects involving unpaid and semi-paid volunteers helping carers. In relationships which are not perceived as purely economic exchanges or where there is a lack of bureaucratic control and hierarchy, there are few boundaries and the demands of the relationship may very easily expand to 'fill the space available'. Volunteer projects in particular can all too quickly reproduce rather than reduce the stresses and strains of informal care by transferring them from the carer to the substitute helper. Clarity in roles and tasks helps to provide boundaries in a relationship for which there are no clear rules and in which expectations and attachments may quickly grow (Qureshi et al., 1987; Leat, 1990).

In addition to clarity in roles and tasks for workers and volunteers there should also be clarity in the role and responsibilities of the management committee. Problems in the distinction between the spheres of authority and responsibility of management committees and officers are inherent in voluntary organisations. There are no easy formulae to resolve this issue but it is one which must be addressed.

Management committees must also have the right mix of skills and experience as well as being willing to manage and take responsibility. Carer-run projects and self-help groups may experience particular difficulties in this area leading ultimately to failure of the project (Hills, 1991). 'Changing from a self-help group to a management board proved difficult, because it necessitated a massive upheaval in the relationships between members, which then led to disruption and conflict' (Haffenden, 1991, p. 78; Handy, 1989). Difficulties arising from major changes in the role and responsibilities of voluntary management committees are especially likely when the organisation is expanding rapidly, handling larger amounts of money, employing workers for the first time or embarking on contracting.

Some projects suffer from too little management, but in others workers and volunteers may have too many managers to whom they are expected to report. There is a strong argument for overall responsibility to be vested in one person so that the worker does not suffer from the stresses and confusion of multiple accountability and knows that support is readily available from a manager who has special responsibility for him/her (Hadley et al., 1984). Case management and contracting are likely to increase the risk of multiple accountability and both case managers and project managers will need to pay particular attention to this issue.

The job of organiser/manager of a new project for carers is likely to be a complex mixture of publicising the project, organising, co-ordinating, liaising with existing funders and at the same time securing further funding, securing cooperation and referrals from professionals, keeping in contact with other voluntary and statutory organisations as well as supporting staff and volunteers. Whether it is possible to find all of these skills in one person and whether it is reasonable to expect any one person to carry out all of these tasks requires discussion. At the very least projects should ensure that they have adequate clerical and administrative support – even if this does not sit easily with their desire to spend as little as possible on administration (Haffenden, 1991; Orlik *et al.*, 1991).

Given the other demands on a manager's time, especially in the early stages of a new venture, it is perhaps not surprising that providing support staff and volunteers sometimes takes a back seat – especially when relationships between volunteers and carers seem to be established and going smoothly (Qureshi *et al.*, 1987; Leat, 1990; Moore and Green, 1985). Volunteers are often expected to work by themselves in highly demanding and potentially stressful situations; even when they are working with others they may need considerable support. Because the needs and demands of carers and those they care for change, and because there are, as noted above, no clear boundaries to social exchange, it is important that the relationships, tasks and work-load of volunteers are regularly reviewed Regular reviews are built into work with children, and there is a strong argument for the same procedures being followed with adults (Qureshi *et al.*, 1987; Thornton, 1989; Leat, 1990). Now, and in the future under case-management systems, one of the most important roles of volunteer/project organisers may be to act as a middle-man or buffer between volunteers and users.

Training of volunteers and paid helpers is a contentious issue. In some types of project, it may be argued, training is appropriate; others object to the use of the term training, preferring instead to emphasise preparation (King's Fund, 1987). In some cases workers may need preparation in various practical tasks, information about other help available and procedures for obtaining it and in understanding the problems of carers and those they care for. In some cases workers may need special help in understanding the purpose of the project, especially when the focus is on carers rather than the more obvious needs of those they care for (Moore and Green, 1985; Leat, 1979). Volunteers may also need help in understanding how they can help and in developing realistic standards against which to judge the visible impact of their input (Moore and Green, 1985).

There is some limited evidence suggesting that those who attend preparation sessions provide a better service (Stalker, 1990).

Just as volunteers and paid workers need support, so too do managers performing an often isolated and demanding job frequently with few immediate tangible results for relatively low pay and with an uncertain future (Haffenden, 1991). Whether volunteer management committee members have either the time or the skills and experience to provide this support is debatable.

Good management also requires clear lines of accountability and standards for evaluation. In part accountability and standards for evaluation follow from the points discussed above, in particular from clarity in goals, strategies and roles. Regular monitoring and evaluation are important not only for internal management purposes but also in securing further funding, and will become increasingly important under contracting. Progress reviews and evaluation should involve both helpers and users, and particular attention should be paid to providing for both positive and negative feedback. Getting carers to 'complain' may be more easily achieved in group rather than individual sessions or by use of anonymous comments (Haffenden, 1991). Accountability between workers/volunteers and managers is, or should be, a two-way process and management needs to consider the scope for contracts, disciplinary and grievance procedures which provide for the enforcement of standards and protection of helpers and users alike. Insurance and legal protection for workers and especially for volunteers is often overlooked but is an area of considerable importance and growing concern (SSI, 1990; Leat, forthcoming).

Finally, any genuine commitment to innovation requires willingness on the part of management to welcome success *and* to tolerate failure (Peters and Austin, 1987; Hadley *et al.*, 1984; Jowell, 1991). Mistakes and failure can be as, if not more, instructive as success if, and only if, there are adequate data and time for reflection and dissemination from which others may learn valuable lessons.

All of the above factors in innovation for carers are not once-and-for-all problems. There is a continuing, ongoing need for keeping close to carers, for clarity in goals and strategies, for adaptation to change, for funding and efficient resource allocation, for balancing supply and demand by maintaining referrals and recruiting and supporting adequate numbers of volunteers and for good management. These problems do not go away, although they may change and assume different degrees of difficulty and significance at different stages in the life of a project.

To summarise:
- Confusion and ambiguity in workers' and volunteers' roles and tasks is one cause of failure in new projects.

- There should also be clarity in the role and responsibilities of the management committee.

- Carer-run projects and self-help groups may experience particular management difficulties leading ultimately to failure of the project.

- Even when working with others volunteers may need considerable support and regular review. Managers also require support.

- Monitoring and evaluation are important not only for internal management purposes but also in securing further funding.

Selected reading

Finch, J. (1989) *Family Obligations and Social Change*, Cambridge: Polity Press.

King's Fund Informal Carers Unit (1987) *Taking a Break: A Guide for People Caring at Home*, London: King's Fund.

Kohner, N. (1988) *Caring at Home: A Handbook for People Looking After Someone at Home*, London: King's Fund.

Lewis and Meredith, B. (1988) *Daughters Who Care: Daughters Caring for Mothers at Home*, London: Routledge.

Parker, G. (1992) *With This Body*, Buckingham: Open University.

Perring, C., Twigg, J. and Atkin, K. (1990) *Families Caring for People Diagnosed as Mentally Ill: The Literature Re-examined*, London: HMSO.

Qureshi, H. and Walker, A. (1989) *The Caring Relationship: Elderly People and Their Families*, Basingstoke: Macmillan.

Robinson, J. and Yee, L. (1991) *Focus on Carers: A Practical Guide to Planning and Delivering Community Care Services*, London: King's Fund.

Twigg, J., Atkin, K. and Perring, C. (1990) *Carers and Services: A Review of Research*, London: HMSO.

Twigg, J. and Atkin K. (1993) *Policy and Practice in Informal Care*, Buckingham: Open University.

Ungerson, C. (1987) *Policy is Personal: Sex, Gender and Informal Care*, London: Tavistock.

References

Abrams, P., Abrams, S., Humphrey, R. and Snaith, R. (1986) *Creating Care in the Neighbourhood*, edited by Leat, D., London: Advance.

ACCAS (1991) *Crossroads Care Review* 90/91, Association of Crossroads Care Attendant Schemes, Rugby.

Action for Research into Multiple Sclerosis (1983) *Discovering the Diagnosis of MS* (General Report No 3), Department of Sociology, Brunel University.

Agnew, J. (1987) *Place and Politics: The Geographical Mediation of State and Society*, London: Macmillan.

Allen, Isobel, C. (1983) *Short-Stay Residential Care for the Elderly*, London: Policy Studies Institute.

Allen, I., Hogg, D. and Peace, S. (1992) *Elderly People: Choice, Participation and Satisfaction*, London: Policy Studies Institute.

Arber, S., Gilbert, N. and Evandrou, M. (1988) 'Gender, household composition and receipt of domicilary services by elderly disabled people', *Journal of Social Policy*, 17, 2, 153 175.

Arber, S. and Gilbert, N. (1989) 'Men: the forgotten carers', *Sociology*, 23, 1:111–118.

Arber, S. and Ginn, J. (1990) ' The meaning of informal care: gender and the contribution of elderly people', *Ageing and Society*, 10, 4: 429–454.

Arber, S. and Ginn, J. (1991) *Gender and Later Life: A Sociological Analysis of Resources and Constraints*, London: Sage.

Arber, S. and Ginn, J. (1992) 'In sickness and in health: Care-giving, gender and the independence of elderly people' in Marsh, C. and Arber, S. (eds) *Families and Households: Divisions and Change*, London: Macmillan.

Arber, S. and Ginn, J. (forthcoming) 'Class and caring: A forgotten dimension', *Sociology*.

Armstrong, D. (1983) *The Political Anatomy of the Body*, Cambridge: Cambridge University Press.

Atkin, K. (1991a) 'Health, illness, disability and black minorities: a speculative critique of present day discourse', *Disability, Handicap and Society*, 6, 1, 37–47.

Atkin, K. (1991b) 'Community care in a multi-racial society: incorporating user views', *Policy and Politics*, 19, 3, 159–166.

Atkin, K. and Rollings, J. (1992) 'Informal Care in Asian and Afro-Caribbean Communities: A Literature Review', *British Journal of Social Work*, 22, 405-418.

Atkin, K. (1992) 'Black carers; the forgotten people', *Nursing the Elderly*, 4, 2: 8–10.

Atkinson, F.I. (1992) 'Experiences of informal carers providing nursing support for disabled dependants', *Journal of Advanced Nursing*, 17: 835–40.

Atkinson, F.I. and McHaffie, H.E. (1992) 'A systematic approach to assessing carers' needs and providing nursing support: An evaluation of outcomes', Edinburgh Nursing Research Unit, University of Edinburgh.

Atkinson, S.M. (1986) *Schizophrenia at Home: A Guide to Helping the Family*, New York: New York University Press.

Audit Commission (1986) *Making a Reality of Community Care*, London: HMSO.

Ayer, S. and Alaszewski, A. (1984) *Community Care and the Mentally Handicapped: Services for Mothers and their Mentally Handicapped children*, London: Croom Helm.

Badger, F., Cameron, E. and Evers, H. (1989) 'The nursing auxiliary service and care of elderly patients', *Journal of Advanced Nursing*, 14, 471–477.

Bagguley, P., Mark-Lawson, J., Shapiro, D., Urry, J., Walby, S. and Wardle, A. (1990) *Restructuring: Place, Class and Gender*, London: Sage.

Baldock, J. and Ungerson, C. (1991) 'What d'ya want if you don't want money? – a feminist critique of "paid volunteering"' in Maclean, M. and Groves, D. (eds) *Women's Issues in Social Policy*, London: Routledge.

Baldwin, S. M. (1977) 'Disabled children – counting the costs', *Disability Alliance*, Pamphlet no.8, London.

Baldwin, S. M. (1985) *The Costs of Caring*, London: Routledge and Kegan Paul.

Baldwin, S. M. and Glendinning, C. (1983) 'Employment, women and their disabled children' in Finch, J. and Groves, D. (eds) *A Labour of Love: Women, Work and Caring*, London: Routledge and Kegan Paul.

Baldwin, S. M., Godfrey, C. and Staden, F. (1983) 'Childhood Disablement and Family Incomes', *Epidemiology and Community Health*, 37: 87–195.

Baldwin, S. and Parker, G. (1991) 'Support for informal carers – the role of social security' in Dalley, G. (ed) *Disability and Social Policy*, London: Policy Studies Institute.

Bandana Ahmad (1989) 'Black pain white hurt', *Social Work Today*, 21, 16, 29.

BASW (1990) *Directory of Adult Placement Schemes,* London: BASW.

Baxter, C. (1989) *Cancer support and ethnic minority and migrant work communities,* a summary of a research report commissioned by Cancerlink.

Bayley, M. (1973) *Mental Handicap and Community Care,* London: Routledge and Kegan Paul.

Beardshaw, V. (1988) *Last on the List: Community Services for People with Physical Disabilities,* London: King's Fund Institute.

Bebbington, A. C., Charnley, H., Davies, B.P., Ferlie, E.B., Hughes, M.D. and Twigg, J. (1986) *The Domiciliary Care Project: Meeting the Needs of the Elderly,* Interim Report, PSSRU, Kent.

Bilsborrow, S. (1992) *You Grow Up Fast As Well: Young Carers on Merseyside,* London: Barnardo's.

Blannin, J. (1987) 'Incontinence: men's problems', *Community Outlook,* February.

Blannin, J. (1992) 'Breaking point', *Nursing Times,* 88, 5: 61–4.

Blaxter, M. (1976) *The Meaning of Disability,* London: Heinemann.

Bodkin, C.M., Pigott, T.J. and Mann, J R (1982) 'Financial burdens of childhood cancer', *British Medical Journal,* 284: 1542–4.

Boldy, D. and Kuh, D. (1984) 'Short term care for elderly in residential homes: a research note', *British Journal of Social Work,* 14: 173–5.

Bone, M. and Meltzer, H. (1989) *OPCS Surveys of Disability in Great Britain: Report 3 – the Prevalence of Disability Among Children,* London: HMSO.

Borne, S. and Lewis, E. (1977) 'Doctors despair: a paradox of progress', *Journal of the Royal College of General Practititioners,* 27: 37–9.

Bowes, A. and Sim, D. (1991) *Demands and Constraints: Ethnic Minorities and Social Services in Scotland,* Edinburgh: SCVO.

Bowling, A. (1984) 'Caring for the elderly widowed: the burden on their supporters', *British Journal of Social Work,* 14, 5: 435–55.

Bradshaw, J. and Lawton, D. (1976) 'Tracing the causes of stress in families with handicapped children', *British Journal of Social Work,* 8, 2: 181–192.

Bradshaw, J. (1980), *The Family Fund: An Initiative in Social Policy,* London: Routledge and Kegan Paul.

Braithwaite, V.A. (1990) *Bound to Care,* Sydney: Allen and Unwin.

Brearley, P. and Mandelstram, M. (1992) *A Review of Literature 1986–1991 on Day Care Services for Adults,* London: HMSO.

Briggs, A. and Oliver, J. (1985) *Caring: Experiences of looking after Disabled Relatives*, London: Routledge and Kegan Paul.

Brisenden, S. (1987) 'A response to physical disability and beyond: a report of the Royal College of Physicians', *Disability, Handicap and Society*, 2, 2: 175–82.

Brocklehurst, J.C. and Tucker, J.S. (1980) *Progress in Geriatric Day Care*, London: King's Fund.

Brody, Elaine M. (1981) '"Women in the Middle" and Family Help to Older People', *The Gerontologist*, 21, 5: 471–80.

Buckquet, D. and Curtis, S. (1986) 'Socio-demographic variation in perceived illness and the use of primary care', *Social Science and Medicine*, 23: 737–44.

Bulmer, M. (1986) *Neighbours: the Work of Philip Abrams*, Cambridge: Cambridge University Press.

Burton, L. (1975) *The Family Life of Sick Children*, London: Routledge and Kegan Paul.

Bury, M. (1982) 'Chronic illness as biographical disruption', *Sociology of Health and Illness*, 4: 167–82.

Byrne, D. G. and White, H. M. (1983) 'State and trait anxiety correlates of illness behaviour in survivors of mycardial infraction', *International Journal of Psychosomatic Medicine*, 13, 1: 1–11.

Byrne, E. A. and Cunningham, C.C. (1985) 'The effects of mentally handicapped children on families', *Journal of Child Psychology and Psychiatry*, 26, 6: 847–64.

Cameron, E., Badger, F. Evers, H. and Atkin, K. (1989) 'Black old women, disability and health carers' in Jeffreys, M. (ed) *Growing Old in the Twentieth Century*, London: Routledge.

Carr, J (1976), 'Effect on the family of a child with Downs Syndrome', *Physiotherapy*, 62, 1: 20–23.

Carr-Hill, R. and Harbajan Chadha-Boreham (1988) 'Racism and welfare: education' in Ashok Bhatt, Carr-Hill, R. and Sushel Ohri (eds), *Britain's Black Population*, Aldershot: Gower.

Carter, J. (1981) *Day Services for Adults: Somewhere to Go*, London: Allen and Unwin.

Cartwright, A., Hockey, L. and Anderson, J.L. (1973) *Life Before Death*, London: Routledge and Kegan Paul.

Cartwright, A. and O'Brien, M. (1976) 'Social class variation in health care and in the nature of general practice consultations' in Stacey, M. (ed) *The*

Sociology of the National Health Service, Sociological Review Monograph No 22, Keele: University of Keele.

Challis, D. and Davies, B. (1985) 'Long term care for the elderly: the Community Care Scheme', *British Journal of Social Work,*15, 6, 563–579.

Challis, D. and Davies, B. (1986) *Case Management in Community Care,* Aldershot: Gower.

Challis, D. and Davies, B. (1991) 'A rejoinder: improving support to carers: a considered response to Parker's critical review', *Ageing and Society,* 11, 69–73.

Challis, D. and Ferlie, E. (1986) 'Changing patterns of fieldwork organisations: the headquarters' view' *British Journal of Social Work,* 16, 181–202.

Challis, D. and Ferlie, E. (1987) 'Changing patterns of fieldwork organisation: the team leaders' view', *British Journal of Social Work,* 17, 147–67.

Challis, D. and Ferlie, E. (1988) 'The myth of general practice: specialisation in social work', *Journal of Social Policy,* 17, 1–22.

Challis, D., Chessum, R., Chesterman, J., Luckett, R. and Woods, B. (1988) 'Community Care for the Frail Elderly: an Urban Experiment', *British Journal of Social Work,* 18, supplement: 13–42.

Charlesworth, A, Wilkin, D. and Durie, A. (1983) *Carers and Services: a Comparison of Men and Women Caring for Dependent Elderly People,* Manchester: University of Manchester, Departments of Psychiatry and Community Medicine.

Chetwynd, J. (1985) 'Factors contributing to stress on mothers caring for an intellectually handicapped child', *British Journal of Social Work,* 15: 295–304.

Clarkson, S.E., Clarkson, J.E., Dittmer, I.E., Flett, R., Linsell, C., Mullen, P. and Mullin, B. (1986) 'Impact of a handicapped child on mental health of parents', *British Medical Journal,* 293: 1395–97.

Connolly, N. (1988) *Caring in the Multi-racial Community,* London: Policy Studies Institute.

Cooke, K. (1982) *1970 Birth Cohort – 10 Year Follow-up Study: Interim Report,* Social Policy Research Unit Working Paper, University of York.

Craig, J. (1983) 'The growth of the elderly population', *Population Trends,* no. 32, London: OPCS.

Creer, C. and Wing, J. K. (1974) *Schizophrenia at Home,* Surbiton: National Schizophrenia Fellowship.

Creer, C. (1975) 'Living with schizophrenia', *Social Work Today,* 6: 2–7.

131

Creer, C., Sturt, E. and Wykes, T. (1982) 'The role of relatives' in Wing, J. K. (ed) 'Long-term community care experience in a London borough', *Psychological Medicine*, 12, monograph supplement 2, 29–39.

Cypher, J. (1988) *Developing Social Services for Ethnic Minority Groups: Overview Report of an Inspection of 3 West Midlands Social Services Department*, London: Social Services Inspectorate, Department of Health.

Dalley, G. (1988) *Ideologies of Caring: Rethinking Community and Collectivism*, London: Macmillan.

Dant, T. and Gearing, B. (1990) 'Keyworkers for elderly people in the Community: case managers and care co-ordinators', *Journal of Social Policy*, 19, 3, 331–360.

Davies, B. (1968) *Social Needs and Resources in Local Services*, London: Michael Joseph.

Davies, B. and Challis, D. (1986) *Matching Resources to Needs in Community Care*, Aldershot: Gower.

Davies, B.P. and Bebbington, A.C. (1983) 'Equity and efficiency in the allocation of personal social services', *Journal of Social Policy*, 12, 3, 309–329.

Department of Health (DH) (1990) *Community Care in the Next Decade and Beyond: Policy Guidance*, London: HMSO.

Dexter, M. and Herbert, W. (1983) *The Home Help Service*, London: Tavistock.

Dingwall, R., Rafferty, A. M. and Webster, C. (1988) *An Introduction to the Social History of Nursing*, London: Routledge.

Dominelli, L. (1989) 'An uncaring profession? An examination of racism in social work', *New Community*, 15, 3, 391–403.

Donaldson, C., Clark, K., Gregson, B., Blackhouse, M. and Pragnal, C. (1988) *Evaluation of a Family Support Unit for Elderly Mentally Infirm People and their Carers*, Newcastle upon Tyne: University of Newcastle upon Tyne, Health Care Research Unit, Report No 34.

Donovan, J. (1986) *We don't buy sickness, it just comes*, Aldershot: Gower Press.

Dunnell, K. and Dobbs, J. (1982) *Nurses Working in the Community*, London: OPCS.

Ellard, J. (1974) 'The disease of being a doctor', *Medical Journal of Australia*, 2: 318–22.

Equal Opportunities Commission (1980) *The Experience of Caring for Elderly and Handicapped Dependants: Survey Report*, Manchester: EOC.

Equal Opportunities Commission (1982) *Caring for the Elderly and Handicapped: Community Care Policies and Women's Lives*, Manchester: EOC.

Evandrou, M., Arber, S., Dale, A. and Gilbert, G. N. (1986) 'Who cares for the elderly: family care provision and receipt of statutory services' in Phillipson, C., Bernard, M. and Strang, P. (eds) *Dependency and Interdependency in Old Age*, London: Croom Helm.

Evandrou, M. (1990) *Challenging the Invisibility of Carers: Mapping Informal Care Nationally*, Discussion Paper WSP/49, STICERD, London School of Economics.

Evans, N., Kendall, I., Lovelock, R. and Powell, J. (1986) *Something to Look Forward to: An Evaluation of a Travelling Day Hospital for Elderly Mentally Ill People*, Portsmouth: SPRIU.

Evers, H., Badger, F., Cameron, E. and Atkin, K. (1988) *The Home Help Service, Elderly and Disabled People*, Birmingham: Health Service Research Centre, University of Birmingham.

Evers, H., Badger, F., Cameron, E. and Atkin, K. (1989) *Community Care Project Working Papers*, Birmingham: Department of Social Medicine, University of Birmingham.

Fadden, G., Bebbington, P. and Kuipers, L. (1987a) 'The burden of care: the impact of functional psychiatric illness on the patient's family', *British Journal of Psychiatry*, 150, 285–292.

Fadden, G., Bebbington, P. and Kuipers, L. (1987b) 'Caring and its burdens: a study of relatives of depressed patients', *British Journal of Psychiatry*, 150, 660–667.

Falek, A. (1979) 'Observations on patient and family coping with Huntington's Disease', *Omega*, 10: 35–42.

Faloon, I.R.H., Boyd, J.L., McGill, G.W., Razani, J., Moos, H.B. and Gilderman, A.M. (1982) 'Family management in the prevention of exacerbations of schizophrenia: a controlled study', *New England Journal of Medicine*, 306, 437–40.

Fennell, G., Emerson, A.R., Sidell, M. and Hague, A. (1981) *Day Centres for the Elderly in East Anglia*, Norwich: Centre for East Anglian Studies.

Fennell, G., Philipson, C. and Evers, H. (1988) *The Sociology of Old Age*, Milton Keynes: Open University Press.

Fenton, S. (1987) *Ageing Minorities: Black People As They Grow Old in Britain*, London: Commission for Racial Equality.

Ferlie, E., Pahl, J. and Quine, L. (1984) 'Professional collaboration in services for mentally handicapped people', *Journal of Social Policy*, 13, 3: 185–202.

Finch, J. and Groves, D. (1980), 'Community care and the family: a case for equal opportunities', *Journal of Social Policy*, 9, 4: 487–511.

Finch, J. and Groves, D. (1983) *A Labour of Love: Women, Work and Caring*, London: Routledge and Kegan Paul.

Fitzpatrick, R. (1984) *The Experience of Illness*, London: Tavistock Publications.

Flynn, M. (1986) *Respite Care: A Review of the Literature*, Ilford: Barnardo's Research and Development.

Forster, A. (1985) 'How to start a support group for relatives looking after a dementia sufferer' in Osborn, A. (ed) *Reaching Out to Dementia Sufferers and Their Carers*, Age Concern Scotland.

Frank, L. (1984) *Respite Care for the Elderly: Some Organisational and Planning Issues*, proceedings of Australian Association of Gerontology, 19th Conference, Sydney 1984.

Friedson, E. (1970) *Profession of Medicine: A Study of the Sociology of Applied knowledge*, New York: Mead and Co.

Further Education Unit (1990) *Self-Advocacy and Parents: The Impact of Self-Advocacy on the Parents of Young People with Disabilities*, London: FEU.

Gibbon, P. (1992) 'Equal opportunity policy and race equality' in Braham, P., Ali Rattansi and Skellington, R. (eds) *Racism and Anti-Racism: Inequalities, Opportunities and Policies*, London: Sage.

Gibbons, J.S., Horn, S.M., Powell, J.M. and Gibbons, J.L. (1984) 'Schizophrenic patients and their families: a survey in a psychiatric service based on a DGH unit', *British Journal of Psychiatry*, 144, 70–77.

Gilhooly, M. (1984) 'The impact of caregiving on caregivers: factors associated with the psychological well-being of people supporting a dementing relative in the community', *British Journal of Medical Psychology*, 57: 35–44.

Gilhooly, M. (1986) 'Senile dementia: factors associated with caregivers' preference for institutional care', *British Journal of Medical Psychology*, 59: 165–71.

Gilleard, C.J., Watt, G. and Boyd, W.D. (1981) 'Problems of caring for the elderly mentally infirm at home', paper presented at the Twelfth International Congress of Gerontology, July 12th–17th, Hamburg, W. Germany.

Gilleard, C.J., Gilleard, E., Gledhill, K. and Whittick, J. (1984) 'Caring for the elderly mentally infirm at home: a survey of the supporters', *Journal of Epidemiology and Community Health*, 38: 319–25.

Gledhill, K.J., Mackie, J.E. and Gilleard, C.J. (1982) 'A comparison of problems and coping reported by supporters of elderly day hospital patients with similar ratings provided by nurses', paper presented to the British Psychological Society Annual Conference, April 1982.

Glendinning, C. (1983) *Unshared Care*, London: Routledge and Kegan Paul.

Glendinning, C. (1985) *A Single Door*, London: George Allen and Unwin.

Glendinning, C. (1992) *The Costs of Informal Care: Looking Inside the Household*, London: HMSO.

Glew, J. (1986) 'Continence a woman's lot?', *Nursing Times*, 9 April.

Glosser, G. and Wexler, D. (1985) 'Participants' evaluation of education-al/support groups for families of patients with Alzheimer's Disease and other dementias', *The Gerontologist*, 25, 3: 323–6

Goddard, J. and Rubissow, J. (1977), 'Meeting the needs of handicapped children and their families. The evolution of Honeylands: a family sup-port unit, Exeter', *Child: Care, Health and Development*, 3: 261–73.

Goldberg, E.M. and Warburton, R.W. (1979) *Ends and Means in Social Work*, London: Allen and Unwin.

Goldman, H. (1980) 'The post hospital mental patient and family therapy', *The Journal of Marital and Family Therapy*, 6, 447–52.

Goodwin, S. (1988) 'Whither health visiting?', *Health Visitor*, 61,12: 379–83.

Grad, J. and Sainsbury, P. (1963) 'Mental illness and the family', *Lancet*, i, 544–47.

Graham, H. (1983) 'Caring: labour of love' in Finch, J. and Groves, D. (eds) *A Labour of Love: Women, Work and Caring*, London: Routledge and Kegan Paul.

Graham, H. (1991) 'The concept of caring in feminist research: the case of domestic service', *Sociology*, 25,1: 61–78.

Graham, J. (1984) Take up of FIS: *Knowledge, Attitudes and Experience – Claimants and Non-Claimants*, Stormont: PPRU.

Green, H. (1988) *General Household Survey 1985: Informal Carers*, London: HMSO.

Griffiths, R. (1988) *Community Care: an Agenda for Action*, London: HMSO.

Grimshaw, R. (1992) *Children of Parents with Parkinson's Disease: A Research Report for the Parkinson's Disease Society*, London: National Children's Bureau.

Gubman, G.D. and Tessler, R.C. (1987) 'The impact of mental illness on families' concepts and priorities', *Journal of Family Issues*, 8, (2 June), 226–45.

Haffenden, S. (1991) *Getting It Right For Carers*, London: HMSO.

Hagan, T. (1989) *Evaluation of Incontinence Training Packages: Final Report*, Social Policy Research Unit, University of York.

Handy, C. (1988) *Understanding Voluntary Organisations*, Penguin Books.

Hasselkus, B.R. and Brown, M. (1983) 'Respite care for community elderly', *American Journal of Occupational Therapy*, 37, 2: 83–8.

Hasselkus, B.R. and Brown, M. (1983) *The Forgotten Army: Family Care and Elderly People*, London: Family Policy Studies Centre.

Herding, J. M. and Modell, M. (1985) 'How patients manage asthma', *Journal of the Royal College of General Practitioners*, 35: 226–8.

Hills, D. (1991) *Carer Support in the Community: Evaluation of the Department of Health Initiative; Demonstration Districts for Informal Carers 1986–1989*, London: HMSO.

Hinrichsen, G.A., Revenson, T.A. and Shinn, G. (1987) 'Does self-help help? An empirical investigation of scoliosis peer support group', *Journal of Social Issues*, 41, 1: 65–87.

Hirst M. A. (1982), *Young Adults with Disabilities and their Families*, Social Policy Research Unit, University of York.

Hirst, M.A. (1983) 'Evaluating the malaise inventory: An item analysis', *Social Psychiatry*, 18: 181–84.

Hirst, M. A. and Bradshaw, J.R. (1983) 'Evaluating the malaise inventory: A comparison of measures of stress', *Journal of Psychosomatic Research*, 27: 193–99.

Hirst, M. A. (1984) *Moving On: Transfer from Child to Adult services for Young People with Disabilities*, Social Policy Research Unit, University of York.

Hirst, M. A. (1992) 'Employment patterns of mothers with a disabled young person', *Work, Employment and Society*, 6, 1: 87–101.

Hopper and Roberts (undated) *Crossroads Care Attendant Schemes*, London: Greater London Association for the Disabled.

Horton, C. and Berthoud, R. (1990) *The Attendance Allowance and Costs of Caring*, London: Policy Studies Institute.

Hubert, J. (1990) 'At home and alone: families and young adults with challenging behaviour' in Booth, T. (ed) *Better Lives: Changing Services for People with Learning Difficulties*, Sheffield: Joint Unit for Social Services Research/Community Care.

Hughes, R. (1986) Social Services for Ethnic Minorities – *Policy and Practice in the North West*, Manchester: DHSS, Social Services Inspectorate.

Hughes, R. and Reba Bhaduri (1987) *Race and Culture in Social Services Delivery: A Study in three Social Services Departments of North West England,* Manchester: DHSS, Social Services Inspectorate.

Hunter, D.J., McKeganey, N.P. and MacPherson, I.A. (1988) *Care of the Elderly: Policy and Practice,* Aberdeen: Aberdeen University Press.

Huntingdon, J. (1981) *Social Work and General Medical Practice,* London: Allen and Unwin.

Hyman, M. (1977) *The Extra Costs of Disabled Living,* London: DIG/ARC.

Illsley, R. (1977) *Review Paper in Health and Health Policy: Priorities for Research,* Report of an Advisory Panel to the Research Initiatives Boards, London.

Ineichen, B., Hall, V. and Russell, O. (1980) *Mental Handicap and Family Needs,* Bristol: Department of Mental Health, University of Bristol, Research Report.

Isaacs, B., Livingston, M. and Neville, Y. (1972) *Survival of the Unfittest: A Study of Geriatric Patients in Glasgow,* London: Routledge and Kegan Paul.

Jaehnig, W. (1979) 'A family service for the mentally handicapped', *Fabian Society Tract,* no. 460, London: Fabian Society.

Jewson, N. D. (1976) 'The disappearence of the sick-man from medical cosmologies 1770–1870, *Sociology,* 10: 225–339.

Johnstone, E.C., Owens, D.G.C., Gold, A., Crow, T.J. and MacMillan, J.F. (1984) 'Schizophrenic patients discharged from hospital – a follow-up study', *British Journal of Psychiatry,* 145, 586–90.

Jones, D.A. and Vetter, N.J. (1984) 'A survey of those who care for the elderly at home: their problems and their needs', *Social Science and Medicine,* 19, 5: 511–14.

Jones, N. (1988) *A Report to the Department on the Attitudes of Older Carers of Mentally Handicapped Adults Living in the Borough,* Hammersmith and Fulham Social Service Department.

Joshi, H. (1987) 'The cost of caring', in Glendinning, C. and Millar, J., (eds) *Women and Poverty,* Brighton: Wheatsheaf Books.

Jowell, T. (1990) in *Care in the Community: Making it Happen,* report on a series of conferences held in March, April and May 1990, London: Department of Health.

Keegan, M. (1984) 'A day centre for the elderly mentally infirm' in Isaacs, B. and Evers, H. (eds) *Innovations in the Care of the Elderly,* London: Croom Helm.

Kelson, N. (1985) *The Short Term Care Project, Eastern Counties,* London: Parkinson's Disease Society.

Kestenbaum, A. (1990) *Use Made of ILF Awards – Pilot Survey*, February, unpublished paper.

King's Fund Discussion Paper (1987) *Family Based Respite Care for Children with a Disability*, London: King's Fund Centre.

Kinsella, G.J. and Duffy, F.D. (1979) 'Psychosocial readjustment in the spouses of aphasic patients', *Scandinavian Journal of Rehabilitation Medicine*, 11: 129–32.

Kiple, K.F. and King, V.I.H. (1981) *Another Dimension to the Black Diaspora*, Cambridge: Cambridge University Press.

Kivett, V. R. and Maxheamuer, R. (1980) 'Perspectives on the childless rural elderly: a comparative analysis', *The Gerontologist*, 20, 6: 708.

Knapp, M. (1990) *Care in the Community: Making It Happen*, report on a series of conferences held in March, April and May 1990, London: Department of Health.

Kramer, R. (1981) *Voluntary Agencies in the Welfare State*, University of California Press.

Kreisman, D. and Joy, V. (1974) 'Family response to the mental illness of a relative: a review of the literature', *Schizophrenia Bulletin*, 10, (7a 11), 34–57.

Kuipers, L. (1979) 'Expressed emotion: a review', *British Journal of Social and Clinical Psychology*, 18, 237–43.

Kuipers, L. (1987) 'Depression and the family' in Orford, J. (ed) *Coping with Disorder in the Family*, London: Croom Helm.

Land, H. and (1978) 'Who cares for family', *Journal of Social Policy*, 7, 3: 257–84.

Land, H. and Rose, H. (1985) 'Compulsory altruism for some or an altruistic society for all' in Bean, P., Ferris, J. and Whynes, D. (eds) *In Defence of Welfare*, London: Tavistock.

Leat, D. (1979) *A Home From Home? Report of a Study of Short-term Family Placement Schemes for the Elderly*, Mitcham: Age Concern England Research Unit.

Leat, D., Tester, S. and Unell, J. (1986) *A Price Worth Paying? A study of the effects of government grant aid to voluntary organisations*, London: Policy Studies Institute.

Leat, D. and Gay, P. (1987) *Paying for Care: An exploratory study of the issues raised by paid care schemes*, London: Policy Studies Institute.

Leat, D. (1988) *Accountability and Voluntary Organisations*, London: NCVO.

Leat, D. (1990) *For Love and Money: the role of payment in encouraging the provision of care*, York: Joseph Rowntree Foundation.

Leat, D. (1979) *Limited Liability? A report on some good neighbour schemes*, Berkhamsted: The Volunteer Centre UK.

Lee, G. R. and Ihinger-Tallman, M. (1980) 'Sibling interaction and morale: the effects of family relations on older people', *Research on Ageing*, 2, 8: 367–391.

Levin, E., Sinclair, I. and Gorbach, P. (1985) 'The effectiveness of the home help service with confused old people and their families', *Research, Policy and Planning*, 3, 2.

Levin, E., Sinclair, I. and Gorbach, P. (1989) *Families, Services and Confusion in Old Age*, Aldershot: Gower.

Levin, E. and Moriarty, J. (1990) *'Ready to Cope again': Sitting, Day and Relief Care for the Carers of Confused Elderly People*, London: National Institute for Social Work.

Lewis, J. and Meredith, B. (1988) *Daughters Who Care: Daughters Caring for Mothers at Home*, London: Routledge and Kegan Paul.

Lightfoot, J. (1992) *Report on an exploratory study of establishment setting and review for district nursing and health visiting*, Social Policy Research Unit, University of York.

Lovelock, R. (1985) 'Health and illness' in Burgess, R.G. (ed) *Key Variables in Social Investigation*, London: Routledge and Kegan Paul.

Luker, K.A. (1979) 'Health visiting and the elderly', *Midwife, Health Visitor and Community Nurse*, 15, 11: 457–9.

Lunn, T. (1990) 'A new awareness', *Community Care*, 22 February.

McCalman, J. (1990) *The Forgotten People*, London: King's Fund Centre.

McGrath, M. and Grant, G. (1992) 'Supporting "needs-led" services: impli cations for planning and management systems', *Journal of Social Policy*, 21, 1: 71–98.

McLaughlin, E. (1991) *Social Security and Community Care: The Case of the Invalid Care Allowance*, London: HMSO.

Marsden, D. and Abrams, S. (1987) 'Allies, liberators, intruders and cuck-oos in the nest: towards a sociology of caring over the life cycle' in Keil, T. (ed) *Women and the Life Cycle*, London: Macmillan.

Martin, J. and White A. (1988), *The Financial Circumstances of Disabled Adults Living in Private Households*, London: HMSO.

Martin, J., White, A. and Meltzer, H. (1989) *Disabled Adults: Services, Transport and Employment*, London: HMSO.

Mayer, J. E. and Timms, N. (1970) *The Client Speaks: Working Class Impressions of Casework*, London: Routledge and Kegan Paul.

Mechanic, D. (1970) 'Correlates of frustration among British general practitioners', *Journal of Social Behaviour*, 11, 2: 87–104.

Meethan, K. (1990) *Voluntary Action in Brighton Neighbourhood Associations*, unpublished PhD Thesis, University of Sussex.

Meethan, K. and Thompson, C. (1991) *Negotiating Community Care: Politics, Localities and Resources*, paper presented to Social Policy Association Annual Conference, Nottingham.

Meethan, K. and Thompson, C. (1992) 'The Scarcroft Project: Interim Report', Social Policy Research Unit, University of York.

Meredith, H. (1990) *Young Carers*, London: Carers National Association.

Meredith, H. (1992) 'Supporting the young carer', *Community Outlook*, May, 15–18.

Moore, J. and Green, J.M. (1985) 'The contribution of voluntary organisations to the support of caring relatives', *Quarterly Journal of Social Affairs*, 1, 2.

Moroney, R. M. (1976) *The Family and the State: Considerations for Social Policy*, London: Longman.

Morris, J. (1991) *Pride Against Prejudice: Transforming Attitudes to Disability*, London: Womens' Press.

Mumma, C. and McCorkle, R. (1982) 'Causal attribution and life threatening disease', *International Journal of Psychosomatic Medicine*, 12: 311–19.

Murphy, E. (1985) 'Day care: who and what is it for?', *New Age*, 31, 7–9.

NAHA (1988) *Action not Words: A Strategy to Improve Health Services for Black and Minority Ethnic Groups*, National Association of Health Authorities.

Nissel, M. and Bonnerjea, L. (1982) *Family Care of the Handicapped Elderly: Who Pays?*, London: Policy Studies Institute.

Nolan, M.R. and Grant, G. (1989) 'Addressing the needs of informal carers: a neglected area of nursing practice', *Journal of Advanced Nursing*, 14: 950–61.

Norman, A. (1980) *Rights and Risks*, London: National Corporation for the Care of Old People.

Norman, A. (1985) *Triple Jeopardy: Growing Old in a Second Homeland*, Policy Studies in Ageing No 3, London: Centre for Policy on Ageing.

Oddy, M., Humphrey, M. and Uttley, D. (1978) 'Stresses upon the relatives of head injured patients', *British Journal of Psychiatry*, 133: 507–13.

Oliver, M. (1987) *Some Reflections on Disabling Services*, unpublished paper presented to Further Education Unit Conference, Thames Polytechnic.

Oliver, M. (1990) *The Politics of Disablement*, London: Macmillan.

O'Neil, A. (1988) *Young Carers: The Tameside Research*, Tameside: Tameside Metropolitan Council.

Ong, B.N. (1991) 'Researching needs in district nursing', *Journal of Advanced Nursing*, 16: 638–47.

Onyett, S. (1992) *Case Management in Mental Health*, London: Chapman and Hall.

OPCS (1984) *Census 1981: Key Statistics for Local Authorities: Great Britain*, London: HMSO.

Orlik, C., Robinson, C. and Russell, O. (1991) *A Survey of Family Based Respite Care Schemes in the United Kingdom*, Bristol: National Association for Family Based Respite Care.

Osmond, R. (1992) *Squaring the Circle*, London: King's Fund Centre.

Oswin, M. (1984) *They Keep Going Away: A Critical Study of Short-Term Residential Care Services for Children Who are Mentally Handicapped*, King Edward's Hospital Fund for London.

Packwood, T. (1980) 'Supporting the family: a study of the organisation and implications of the hospital provision of holiday relief for families caring for dependants at home', *Social Science and Medicine*, 14a: 613–20.

Page, R. (1988) *Report on the Initial Survey Investigating the Number of Young Carers in Sandwell Secondary School*, Sandwell: Metropolitan Borough Council.

Parker, G. (1985) *With Due Care and Attention: A Review of Research on Informal Care*, (First Edition) London: Family Policy Studies Centre.

Parker, G. (1989) *A Study of Non-Elderly Spouse Carers: Final Report*, Social Policy Research Unit, University of York.

Parker, G. (1990a) *With Due Care and Attention: A Review of Research on Informal Care*, (Second Edition) London: Family Policy Studies Centre.

Parker, G. (1990b) 'Whose care? Whose costs? Whose benefit? A critical review of research on case management and informal care', *Ageing and Society*, 10, 459–467.

Parker, G. and Lawton, D. (1990a) *Further Analysis of the 1985 General Household Survey Data on Informal Care. Report 1: A Typology of Caring*, Social Policy Research Unit, University of York.

Parker, G. and Lawton, D. (1990b) *Further Analysis of the 1985 General Household Survey Data on Informal Care. Report 2: The Consequences of Caring*, Social Policy Research Unit, University of York.

Parker, G. and Lawton, D. (1991a) *Further Analysis of the 1985 General Household Survey Data on Informal Care. Report 3: Carers and Services*, Social Policy Research Unit, University of York.

Parker, G. and Lawton, D. (1991b) *Further Analysis of the 1985 General Household Survey Data on Informal Care. Report 4: Male Carers*, Social Policy Research Unit, University of York.

Parker, G. (1992) *With This Body: Caring and Disability in Marriage*, Buckingham: Open University Press.

Parker, G. and Lawton, D. (forthcoming) *Different Types of Care: Different Types of Carer*, London: HMSO.

Pearson, R.M. (1988) *Social Services in a Multi-racial Society*, Social Services Inspectorate: Department of Health.

Pentol, A. (1983) 'Cost bearing burdens', *Health and Social Service Journal*, 8 September.

Perring, C., Twigg, J. and Atkin, K. (1990) *Families Caring for People Diagnosed as Mentally Ill: The Literature Re-Examined*, London: HMSO.

Peters, T. and Austin, N. (1985) *A Passion for Excellence*, Glasgow: Fontana/Collins.

Phillipson, C. (1982) *Capitalism and the Construction of Old Age*, London: Macmillan.

Platt, S. (1985) 'Measuring the burden of psychiatric illness on the family: an evaluation of some rating scales', *Psychological Medicine*, 15, 2: 383–93.

Prime, R. (1987) *Developing Social Services to Black and Ethnic Minority Elders in London: Overview Report and Action Plan*, London: Department of Health and Social Security, Social Services Inspectorate.

Quine, L. and Pahl, J. (1985) 'Examining the causes of stress in families with severely mentally handicapped children', *British Journal of Social Work*, 15: 501–17.

Quine, L. and Pahl, J. (1989) *Stress and Coping in Families Caring for a Child with Severe Mental Handicap: A Longitudinal Study*, Canterbury: Institute of Social and Applied Psychology and Centre for Health Services Studies, University of Kent.

Qureshi, H. (1986) 'Responses to dependency: reciprocity, effect and power in family relationships' in Phillipson, C., Bardard, M. and Strang, P. (eds) *Dependency and Interdependency in Old Age: Theoretical Perspectives and Policy Alternatives*, Beckenham: Croom Helm.

Qureshi, H., Challis, D. and Davies, B. (1989) *Helpers in Case-Managed Community Care*, Aldershot: Gower.

Qureshi, H. and Walker, A. (1989) *The Caring Relationship: Elderly People and Their Families*, London: Macmillan.

Race, D. (1987) 'Normalisation: theory and practice' in Malin, N. (ed) *Reassessing Community Care*, London: Croom Helm.

Rai, G.S., Bielawska, C., Murphy, P.J. and Wright, G. (1986) 'Hazards for elderly people admitted to respite ("holiday admissions") and social care ("social admissions")', *British Medial Journal*, 22, 25 January.

Rex, J. and Mason, D. (1986) *Theories of Race and Ethnic Relations*, Cambridge: Cambridge University Press.

Richardson, A. and Goodman, M. (1983) *Self-help and Social Care Mutual Aid Organisations in Practice*, London: Policy Studies Institute.

Richardson, A., Unell, J. and Aston, B. (1989) *A New Deal for Carers*, London: Informal Caring Unit, King's Fund Centre.

Richardson, A. and Higgins, R. (1992) *The Limits of Care Management: Lessons from the Wakefield Care Management Project*, Leeds: Nuffield Institltule.

Robinson, C. (1987) 'Key issues for social workers placing children for family based respite care', *British Journal of Social Work*, 17, 3, 257–283.

Robinson, C. (1988) 'Learning to help: training for respite carers', *Social Work Today*, 2 June, 19, 39.

Robinson, C. and Stalker, K. (1992) *New Directions: Suggestions for Interesting Service Development in Respite Care*, King's Fund Centre.

Robinson, J. (1985) 'Health visiting and health' in White, R. (ed) *Political Issues in Nursing: Past, Present and Future*, Chichester: John Wiley.

Robinson, R. (1978) *In Worlds Apart: Professionals and Their Clients in the Welfare State*, London: Bedford Square Press.

Rojek, C., Peacock, G. and Collins, S. (1988) *Social Work and Received Ideas*, London: Routledge.

Rosenbaum, M. and Najenson, T. (1976) 'Changes in life patterns and symptoms of low mood as reported by wives of severely brain-injured soldiers', *Journal of Consulting Clinical Psychology*, 44,6:881–8.

Rowlings, C. (1981) *Social Work with Elderly People*, London: Allen and Unwin.

Roy, R. (1991) 'Consequences of parental illness on children: a review', *Social Work and Social Sciences Review*, 2:2.

Royal College of Physicians (1986) *Physical Disability in 1986 and Beyond*, London: Royal College of Physicians.

Roys, P. (1988) 'Racism and welfare: social services' in Ashok Bhat, Carr-Hill, R. and Sushel Ohri (eds) *Britain's Black Population, A New Perspective*, Aldershot: Gower.

Sanderson, J. (1991) *An Agenda for Action on Continence Services*, London: Department of Health.

Sandwell Caring for Carers Project (1989) *Child Carer Report*, Sandwell Caring for Carers; Sandwell Social Services Department.

Scharlach, A. and Frenzel, C. (1986) 'An evaluation of institution-based respite care', *The Gerontologist*, 26, 1.

Scott, Mike (1988) 'Racism in the fabric', *Social Work Today*, 20, 6, 42.

Seed, P. (1988) *Day Care at the Crossroads*, Tunbridge Wells: Costello.

Shaw, C. (1988) 'Latest estimates of ethnic minority populations', *Population Trends*, 51, 5–8.

Shaw, M. and Hipgrave, T. (1983) *Specialist Fostering Child Care Policy and Practice*, Batsford Academic and British Agencies for Adoption and Fostering.

Sinclair, I. (1988) 'Residential care for elderly people' in Sinclair, I. (ed) *The Research Reviewed (Vol 2 of Wagner Report)*, London: HMSO.

Sinclair, I. (1990) 'Carers: their contribution and quality of life' in Sinclair, I., Parker, R., Leat, D. and Williams, J. (eds) *The Kaleidoscope of Care: A Review of Research of Welfare Provision for Elderly People*, London: HMSO.

Sinclair, I., Parker, R., Leat, D. and Williams, J. (eds) (1990) *The Kaleidoscope of Care: A Review of Welfare Provision for Elderly People*, London: HMSO.

Sines, D. and Bicknell, J. (1985) *Caring for Mentally Handicapped People in the Community*, London: Harper and Row.

Smith, G. and Cantley, C. (1985) *Assessing Health Care: A Study in Organisational Evaluation*, Milton Keynes: Open University Press.

Smyth, M. and Robus, N. (1989) *The Financial Circumstances of Families with Disabled Children Living in Private Households*, London: HMSO.

Social Services Inspectorate (1987a) *Care for a Change? Inspection of Short-Term Care in the Personal Social Services*, London: DHSS.

Social Services Inspectorate (1987b) *From Home Help to Home Care: An Analysis of Policy, Resourcing and Service Management*, London: DHSS.

144

Social Services Inspectorate (1988) *Managing Policy Change in Home Help Services*, London: DHSS.

Social Services Inspectorate (1990) *Reports of an inspection of adult placement schemes in Solihull*, London: DH.

Social Services Inspectorate (1991a) *Care Management and Assessment: Practitioner's Guide*, London: HMSO.

Social Services Inspectorate (1991b) *Care Management and Assessment: Manager's Guide*, London: HMSO.

Social Services Inspectorate (1991c) *Assessment Systems: Community Care*, London: HMSO.

Social Services Inspectorate (1991d) *Getting the Message Across: A Guide to Developing and Communicating Policies, Principles and Procedures on Assessment*, London: HMSO.

Stalker, K. (1990) *'Share the Care': An Evaluation of a Family-Based Respite Care Service*, London: Jessica Kingsley Publishers.

Stimson, G.V. and Webb, B. (1975) *Going to See the Doctor: The Consultation Process in General Practice*, London: Routledge and Kegan Paul.

Tameside Metropolitan Borough Council (1989) *Informal Care Tameside*, Tameside: Tameside Metropolitan Borough Council.

Tester, S. (1989) *Caring by Day: A Study of Day Care Services for Older People*, London: Centre for Policy on Ageing.

Thompson, D.M. and Haran, D. (1985) 'Living with an amputation: The helper', *Social Science and Medicine*, 20 ,4: 319–23.

Thompson, E. H. and Doll, W. (1982) 'The burden of families coping with the mentally ill: an invisible crisis', *Family Relations: Journal of Applied Family and Child Studies*, 35,3: 379–88.

Thornton, P. and Moore, J. (1980) *The Placement of Elderly People in Private Households: An analysis of current provision*, Leeds: University of Leeds, Department of Social Policy and Administration Monograph.

Thornton, P. (1989) *Creating a Break: A Home Care Relief Scheme for Elderly People and Their Supporters*, Mitcham: Age Concern England.

Tinker, A. (1984) *Staying at Home: Helping Elderly People*, London: HMSO.

Titterton, M. (1992) 'Managing threats to welfare: the search for a new paradigm of welfare', *Journal of Social Policy*, 21, 1: 1–23.

Todd, J. and Young, P. (1988) 'Assisted lodgings and family placement schemes' in Baldwin, S., Parker, G. and Walker, R. (eds) *Social Security and Community Care*, Aldershot: Avebury.

Toseland, R.W., Labrecque, M.S., Goebel, S.T. and Whitney, M.H. (1992) 'An evaluation of a group program for spouses of frail elderly veterans', *The Gerontologist*, xx, x, 1–11.

Townsend, P. (1962) *The Last Refuge: A Survey of Residential Institutions and Homes for Aged in England and Wales*, London: Routledge and Kegan Paul.

Townsend, P. (1981) 'The Structured Dependency of the Elderly: A Creation of Social Policy in the Twentieth Century', *Ageing and Society*, 1, 5–28.

Townsend, P. (1981) 'Elderly people with disabilities', in Walker, A. and Townsend, P. (eds) *Disability in Britain: A Manifesto of Rights*, Oxford: Martin Robertson.

Twigg, J. (1988) 'With carers in mind', *Carelink*, Summer, 5.

Twigg, J. (1989a) 'Models of carers: how do social care agencies conceptualise their relationship with informal carers', *Journal of Social Policy*, 18,1, 53–66.

Twigg, J. (1989b) 'Not taking the strain', *Community Care*, 27 July, 16–18.

Twigg, J. (1990) 'Personal care and the interface between the district nursing and home help services' in Davies, B.P., Bebbington, A.C. and Charnley, H. (eds) *Resources and Outcomes*, Aldershot: Gower.

Twigg, J. (1992) 'The interweaving of formal and informal care: policy models and problems' in Evers, A. (ed) *Better Care for Dependent People Living at Home*, Vienna: European Centre.

Twigg, J., Atkin, K. and Perring, C. (1990) *Carers and Services: A Review of Research*, London: HMSO.

Twigg, J. and Atkin, K. (1993) *Policy and Practice in Informal Care*, Buckingham: Open University Press.

Tyne, A. (1982) 'Community care and mentally handicapped people' in Walker, A. (ed) *Community Care: The Family, the State and Social Policy*, Oxford: Basil Blackwell and Martin Robertson.

Ungerson, C. (1983) 'Women and caring: skills, tasks and taboos' in Gamarnikow, D., Morgan, D., Purvis, J. and Taylorson, D. (eds) *The Public and the Private*, London: Heinemann.

Ungerson, C. (1987) *Policy is Personal: Sex, Gender and Informal Care*, London: Tavistock.

Vaughn, C. E. and Leff, I. P. (1981) 'Patterns of emotional response in relatives of schizophrenic patients', *Schizophrenia Bulletin*, 7, 1: 43–4.

Wade, B., Sawyer, L. and Bell, S. (1983) *Dependency with Dignity*, occasional paper on social administration, Bradford Square Press for the National Council for Voluntary Organisation.

Walker, A. (1980) 'The Social Creation of Poverty and Dependency in Old Age', *Journal of Social Policy*, 9, 172–88.

Ward, L. (1990) 'A programme for change: current issues in services for people with learning disabilities' in Booth, T. (ed) *Better Lives: Changing Services for People with Hearing Difficulties*, Sheffield: Joint Unit for Social Services Research/Community Care.

Weaver, T., Willcocks, D. and Kellaher, L. (1985) *The Business of Care: A Study of Private Residential Homes for Old People*, London: CESSA, North London Polytechnic.

Wenger, C. (1984) *The Supportive Network: Coping with Old Age*, London: George Allen and Unwin.

Whitfield, J.S. (1990) *Inspection into the Arrangements made for the Provision of Social Services to People from Minority Ethnic Groups by the SSDs in Bradford, Kirklees, Leeds and Sheffield*, SSI, Yorkshire and Humberside Region, Department of Health.

Wilkin, D. (1979) *Caring for the Mentally Handicapped Child*, London: Groom Helm.

Williams, J. (1990) 'Elders from black and minority ethnic communities' in Sinclair, I., Parker, R., Leat, D. and Williams, J. (eds) *The Kaleidoscope of Care*, London: HMSO.

Williams, R.G.A. (1983) 'Concepts of health: an analysis of lay logic', *Sociology*, 17: 185–205.

Williams, R. (1988) 'The black experience of social services', *Social Work Today*, 19,19, 14–15.

Wilson, E. (1982) 'Women, the "community" and the "family"' in Walker, A. (ed) *Community Care: The Family and Social Policy*, Oxford: Blackwell

Wilson, J. (1986) *Self-Help Groups Getting Started, Keeping Going*, London: Longmans.

Wright, F.D. (1986) *Left to Care Alone*, Aldershot: Gower.

Young, P. (1988) *The Provision of Care in Supported Lodgings and Unregistered Homes*, London: HMSO.

Zarit, S.H. 'Do we need another 'stress and caregiving study?', *The Gerontologist*, 29, 2: 147–8.

Index

General Household Survey (1980) 20, 33
General Household Survey (1985) 6, 8, 9, 11, 16, 17, 19, 20, 27, 28
general practitioners 57, 66
  and identification of hidden carers 117
  support for carers from 70–4
geographical differences in service provision 57–8
geriatricians 75
Ginn, J. 9, 14, 15, 56
goals
  of innovations 111–13
  of visiting schemes 99
guilt 49, 105
  felt by parental carers 32, 43
  felt by spouse carers 31, 45
  overcoming 119

Haffenden, S. 107
health authorities 100, 101, 105
health services 51–2, 70–9
health visitors 79
heavily involved carers 12, 14, 15, 21–2, 26, 27
helpers 14, 98–99
  matching with carers 119–20
  payment of 98, 99, 100, 103, 104, 105, 115–16
  recruitment of 98, 103–4, 105, 112, 116–17
  supply and demand of 105–6, 117, 120–1
  see also volunteers; workers
Hills, D. 107
home care services 67–70
  organisers of 69
  unreliability of 69, 70
home helps 27, 28, 51, 68
  and personal care 69
hospital doctors, contact of with carers 74–6
hospitals
  discharge from 74–5
  respite care in 85, 87
hours of caring 11
household tasks, help with 51, 68
housing 5, 16

impairment, nature of 13–15
incontinence 49, 77–8, 83

independence 19
  for adult disabled children 33–4, 43, 44
  for people with mental health problems 46
  personal support services and 16
  right to 62–3, 64–5
Independent Living Fund (ILF) 102–3
informal care 2, 10, 64
information for carers 45, 50, 106–8
  from GPs 72, 74
  from support groups 89
innovations 59–60, 95–7, 110
  carers' attitude to 119–20
  examples of 96–108
  goals of 111–15
  management of 121–5
  organisers of 117, 119–23
  resources for 113–15
institutional admission 68, 81, 85
intermittent care 84
intervention 23, 24, 26–7, 39, 49–50
invisible carers 48, 71, 75, 113–14, 117
involvement of carers
  level of 14–15, 18, 21
  in planning 108–10

joint carers 12
Jowell, T. 110

Kent Community Care Scheme 91, 99
Kramer, R. 95

labour, needed for development of services 113, 114
Lawton, D. 9, 10
learning disabilities 42–4
  day care for people with 80, 81, 83–4
Levin, E. 67, 68, 71, 72, 75, 77, 85, 86
Lewis, J. 70, 86
lifting 52, 78
local authorities 7, 104

main carers 12, 19
mainstream services 59–60, 65–93
male carers 19, 20–1, 51
management
  of Crossroads schemes 101

visiting (cont.)

   of carers   66
   by GPs   71
voluntary agencies   109, 111
   co-ordination with other services
    111
   and day care   80, 81
   difficulties of reaching carers   118
   and innovation   95–6
volunteers   98, 99, 114, 121–2
   and needs of carers   99
   recruitment of   105, 115–17
   supply and demand of   105–6, 117,
    120–1
   training of   120–1, 123
voucher systems   120

welfare agencies 63–5
Wilson, J.   91
withdrawal of nursing services   77, 78
women   103
   as carers   17, 19–20, 21, 33, 34, 51
   and housework   68
   informal care seen as oppressive to
    51, 52
workers   99
   clarity in role of   121, 122
   in Crossroads schemes   101
   in flexible respite schemes   103,
    104
   recruitment of   116
   training of   123
working-class
   carers from   56, 57
   and need for neighbourhood care
    schemes   98
   recruitment of volunteers from
    112
Wright, F. D.   71

Yorkshire Regional Health Authority
  Carers' Project   62

Printed in the United Kingdom for HMSO.
Dd.0294540, 11/92, C20, 3396/4, 5673, 214622